Transplantation in Practice

Hasan Fattah • Virgilius Cornea
Editors

Transplantation in Practice

Lessons from Common and Complex Kidney Cases

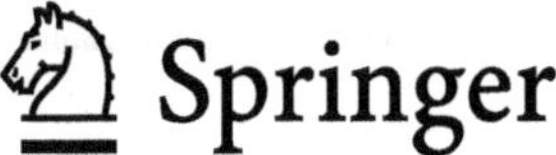

Editors
Hasan Fattah
Jacob School of Medicine and
Biomedical Science
University at Buffalo
Buffalo, NY, USA

Virgilius Cornea
University of Kentucky
Lexington, KY, USA

ISBN 978-3-032-15907-6 ISBN 978-3-032-15908-3 (eBook)
https://doi.org/10.1007/978-3-032-15908-3

This Springer imprint is published by the registered company Springer Nature Switzerland AG
The registered company address is: Gewerbestrasse 11, 6330 Cham, Switzerland

To the mentors and colleagues whose guidance shaped this work.

To the residents and fellows who carry forward the spirit of learning and discovery in transplantation medicine.

To the patients whose resilience and trust continue to teach us the true meaning of healing.

To the University of Kentucky and Jacob School of Medicine and Biomedical Sciences whose academic community and commitment to excellence made this work possible.

To my family, Yasmin, Eyass, Wissam, and Ayser for their unwavering love, patience, and support throughout this journey.

Foreword

Nephrology is considered a difficult topic. Medical students and residents shy away from the specialty and universally opine that renal physiology is a challenging topic. The alchemical ability of the kidneys to turn blood into urine without moving parts is seen as a complex series of nonintuitive functions.

What follows from renal physiology in offering an equally stressful syllabus to the novice is renal pathology. Populated by a novel vocabulary of words and phrases, renal pathology is often considered another disincentive to the study of the kidneys. Further differentiation leads the student to a subset of renal physiology and pathology, that of the kidney transplant. As if the distinction of the anions from the cations, the acids from the bases, was not puzzling enough, transplantology requires the study of immunology as a separate kind of physiology, while separation of the T cells from the B cells is required to understand another kind of pathology.

This intricate set of biological mechanisms is elucidated in a new and remarkably clear manner by Dr. Hasan Fattah in the current volume, *Transplantation in Practice: Lessons from Common and Complex Kidney Cases*. The text meets an important unmet need in the study of kidney transplants. It would not be correct to state that the voluminous content presented here is "simplified," given its elaborateness. But the presentation is so attractively and succinctly made that the reader will find the profusion of information easily understood.

In a series of 10 chapters, each of which consists of several, illustrative cases, Dr. Fattah and colleagues present the salient points of a diverse set of transplant problems. Each case consists of a "*case study summary*," a brief explanation of the "*diagnosis*," a "*management approach*," some "*follow up*," the bullet points of "*educational insights*" and a clinical "*pearl*" which offers a final didactic statement to be incorporated into one's fund of knowledge. One of the most notable features of the format, which really enhances each clinical case's value, is its juxtaposition with a picture of the relevant pathology. The result is that a broad range of 58 different pathologies are brought forth in a most enlightening way. The topics include, to name just a few: T cell-mediated rejection, antibody-mediated rejection, glomerulonephritis, and infection-related kidney injury.

Dr. Fattah is supremely qualified to author this text. Given his extensive training and experience in the transplant field, it's not surprising that he has devised this innovative way of teaching this curriculum. He trained in nephrology at NYU Langone Health and in kidney transplantation at Virginia Commonwealth University. He then went to the University of Kentucky, rising to become Medical Director of the Kidney and Pancreas Transplant Program and Associate Professor of Medicine. Today he is an associate professor in the Transplant Nephrology program at the University at Buffalo, Jacobs School of Medicine and Biomedical Science.

Transplant biology is on the cutting edge of breakthroughs in clinical medicine, with new understandings of immunology and xenobiology occurring right now. In order to address the coming complexity of the resulting medical issues, we need more educational programs to describe it. Dr. Fattah's appealing approach to transplant medicine in this sophisticated new work could be and should therefore be applied to more nephrology topics. It has elucidated the key issues in a wide variety of transplant problems. He has taken up the question of how to make nephrology more comprehensible.

David S. Goldfarb
Professor of Medicine and Physiology
NYU Grossman School of Medicine,
Clinical Chief, Nephrology Division,
NYU Langone Health, Chief, Nephrology
and Medical Director of Hemodialysis,
New York Harbor VA Healthcare System,
New York, NY, USA

Preface

Kidney transplantation remains one of the great achievements in modern medicine, yet the complexity of post-transplant care continues to challenge even experienced clinicians. *Transplantation in Practice: Lessons from Common and Complex Kidney Cases* was conceived to bridge the gap between transplant science textbooks and bedside management by guiding trainees through real-world clinical scenarios.

This book is intended for medical students, internal medicine, surgical residents, nephrology and transplant fellows, and all transplant care providers who are interested and working on developing their understanding of transplantation medicine. Through a case-based approach, it aims to illustrate not only the medical and pathological aspects of kidney transplantation but also the critical thinking, multidisciplinary collaboration, and compassion required to care for transplant recipients.

The cases presented here were drawn from the rich clinical experiences within our academic institutions. Each represents a teaching opportunity to highlight diagnostic reasoning, review evolving evidence, and discuss practical decision-making in the face of complexity.

It is my hope that this work will serve as both a learning tool and a source of reflection for those committed to advancing the field of kidney transplantation and improving patient outcomes.

Buffalo, NY, USA — Hasan Fattah
Lexington, KY, USA — Virgilius Cornea

Acknowledgments

I would like to extend my sincere thanks to Dr. John Tomaszewski for kindly providing some of the case images that helped bring this subject to life. I am also grateful to Dr. Peter Sawaya and Dr. Jon Von Visger for their valuable guidance and advice, and to Dr. David Goldfarb for his mentorship.

Your willingness to share your knowledge and resources is deeply appreciated.

Contents

Contributors

Ana Lia Castellanos Division of Nephrology, Bone and Mineral Metabolism, University of Kentucky, Medical Center, Lexington, KY, USA

Hasan Fattah Jacob School of Medicine and Biomedical Science, University at Buffalo, Buffalo, NY, USA

Sravanthi Paluri Division of Nephrology, Bone and Mineral Metabolism, University of Kentucky, Lexington, KY, USA

Fawad Shuaib Division of Nephrology, Bone and Mineral Metabolism, University of Kentucky, Lexington, KY, USA

Alloimmune Kidney Injury: T Cell-Mediated Rejection (TCMR)

1

Hasan Fattah

Case 1.1

Case Study Summary

Patient: A 27-year-old female with a history of end-stage renal disease (ESRD) secondary to type 1 diabetes mellitus (DM1).

Transplant course: She underwent a 5/6 human leukocyte antigen (HLA) mismatched living-unrelated kidney transplant (LUKT). She is not immunologically sensitized; her calculated panel-reactive antibody (cPRA) was 0%. Induction therapy included antithymocyte globulin (ATG) and steroids; maintenance regimen included tacrolimus-mycophenolate mofetil (tac-mmf) combination and daily prednisone.

Post-transplant Clinical course: Four months after the transplant, mycophenolate mofetil was reduced due to neutropenia, and tacrolimus trough level was kept at a range from 4 to 8 ng/ml. Nine months after the transplant, there was a noted increase in donor-derived cell-free DNA (dd-cfDNA) from 0.06% to 0.9% (>61% change). Additionally, de novo donor-specific antibodies (DSAs) were detected with a total mean fluorescence intensity

H. Fattah (✉)
Jacob School of Medicine and Biomedical Science, University at Buffalo, Buffalo, NY, USA

H. Fattah, V. Cornea (eds.), *Transplantation in Practice*,
https://doi.org/10.1007/978-3-032-15908-3_1

(MFI) of 10,000 against variable class I and class II HLA antigens. Interestingly the creatinine remained stable at a baseline of 1.1 mg/dL, and routine urinalysis showed no active sediments.

Diagnosis

- Moderate to severe T cell-mediated rejection (TCMR) based on molecular diagnostics.
- Acute T cell-mediated rejection (TCMR) grade 1B based on histological examination and Banff 2019 classification (Figs. 1.1 and 1.2).
- No evidence of antibody-mediated rejection (ABMR) on both diagnostic platforms (histology and molecular panels).

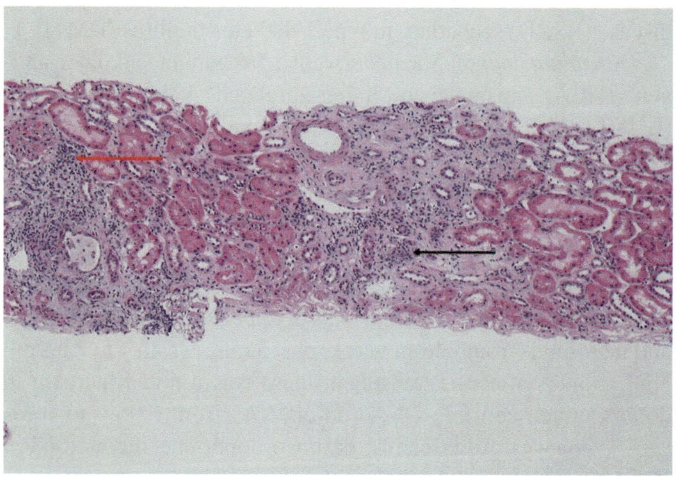

Fig. 1.1 Interstitial lymphatic inflammation (red arrow), and tubulitis (black arrow). H&E. 10X

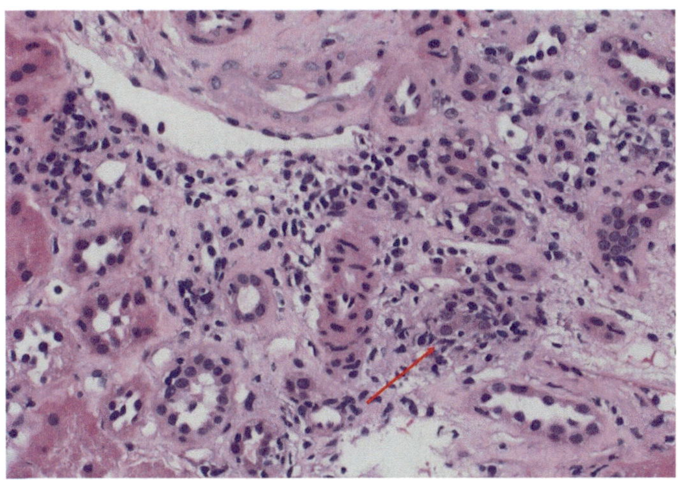

Fig. 1.2 Severe t3 tubulitis (red arrow). H&E, 40× original magnification

Management Approach

Several risk factors may have contributed to the development of rejection in this case, including:

- High degree of HLA mismatch.
- Preemptive reduction in mycophenolate mofetil (MMF) and tacrolimus doses due to side effects.
- Potential noncompliance with immunosuppressive medications.

  Treatment:

- Initiation of ATG therapy and intravenous steroids.
- Adjustment of immunosuppressive therapy, including increasing the baseline immunosuppression agents' levels.

Case Follow-Up

- The patient's creatinine remains stable.
- No evidence of evolving proteinuria on repeated urinalysis at the latest follow-up labs.
- dd-cfDNA has decreased back to 0.1% after treatment.

Educational Insight

- Cellular-mediated rejection may evolve as a subtle disease, especially in living donor kidney young transplant recipients who are at high risk of rejection due to factors such as high HLA mismatch degree and on reduced immunosuppressive doses due to noncompliance or side effects.
- Importance of Serial Molecular Testing: Molecular diagnostics (such as dd-cfDNA testing) may be critical for detecting early complications such as subclinical rejection [1] earlier in high-risk transplant groups, particularly when clinical signs are lacking.
- Differentiating TCMR from Other Forms of Rejection: Unlike antibody-mediated or mixed rejection, TCMR is not associated with significant increase in dd-cfDNA levels. An increase in dd-cfDNA >0.5% from baseline was significantly correlated with clinical and subclinical allograft rejection [2].

Pearl 1.1

This case underscores the importance of vigilant monitoring and the use of molecular diagnostics to detect early rejection in high-risk transplant recipients, particularly when clinical signs are minimal.

Case 1.2

Case Study Summary

Patient: 44-year-old female with medical history of end-stage renal disease (ESRD) secondary to type 2 diabetes mellitus (DM).

Transplant course: she received Living unrelated kidney transplant (LUKT), 4/6 HLA mismatch, calculated PRA (cPRA) was 0%. Post-transplant baseline creatinine 1.2 mg/dl. Immunosuppression included induction treatment with ATG, steroids, followed by maintenance tacrolimus, mycophenolate mofetil (tac-mmf) combination, and daily prednisone.

Post-transplant clinical course:

- Routine follow-up and labs at 18 months. Creatinine increased to 1.6 mg/dL. Urinalysis: no active sediments.
- dd-cfDNA and DSA: both were negative.

Diagnosis

- Pathology diagnosis:
  - Chronic allograft arteriopathy with intimal thickening and vascular changes (Figs. 1.3 and 1.4).
  - Chronic active T cell-mediated rejection (caTCMR) features (Fig. 1.5).
  - No evidence of antibody-mediated rejection (ABMR).
- No evidence of acute rejection based on molecular transcripts Molecular Microscope Diagnostic System (MMDx).

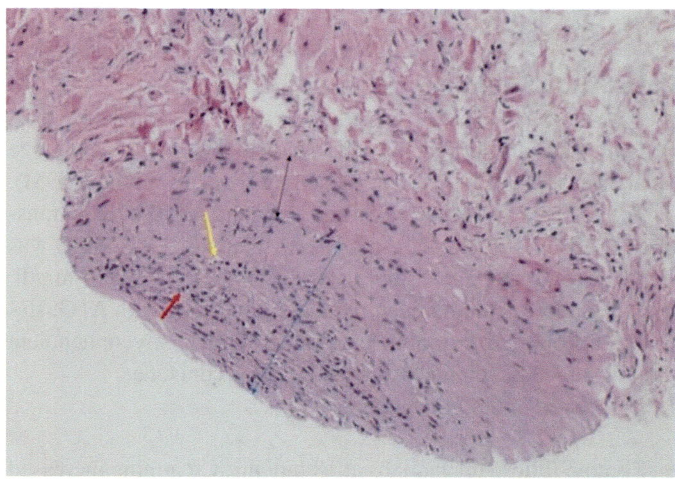

Fig. 1.3 Artery with chronic allograft arteriopathy with neointimal formation and fibrosis (blue arrow), mononuclear cell infiltrate (red arrow), foamy cells (yellow arrow), and arterial media (black arrow). H&E, 20×

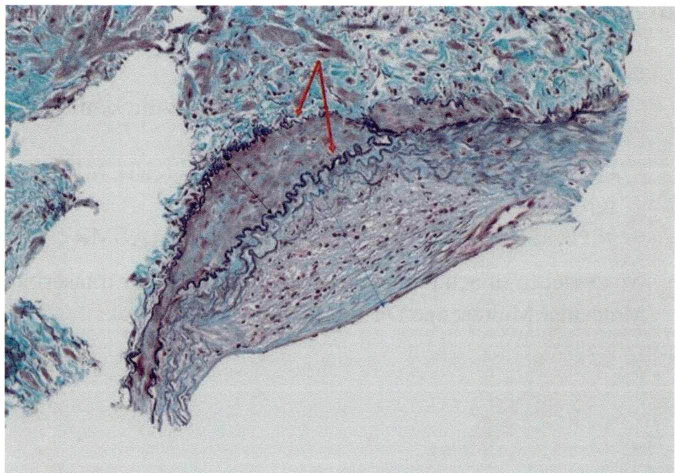

Fig. 1.4 Artery with chronic allograft arteriopathy with neointimal formation and fibrosis (blue arrow), arterial media (black arrow), and elastic laminae (red arrows). Elastic-thricrome stain, 20×

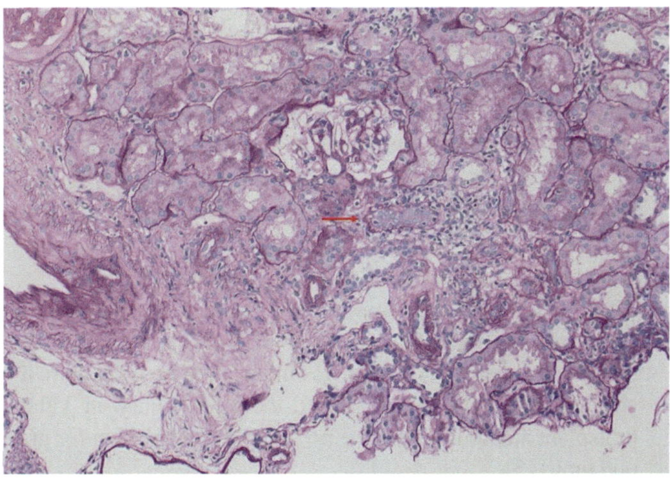

Fig. 1.5 Moderate t2 tubulitis (red arrow) and chronic allograft arteriopathy; this is not specific for either chronic active cellular or humoral rejection; however, the t2 tubulitis in the absence of histologic features of antibody-mediated rejection is supportive of chronic active T cell-mediated rejection. PAS, 20×

Management Approach

- Ensuring compliance and optimizing maintenance immunosuppression.
- Conversion from tacrolimus-based regimen to belatacept to reduce calcineurin inhibitor-related nephrotoxicity and optimize immunosuppressive control.

Case Follow-Up

- Creatinine at 2 years: improved to 1.1 mg/dL. Urinalysis: remains nonactive.
- No recurrence of rejection or proteinuria based on repeat labs and serial ddcfDNA follow-up levels.

Educational Insights

Chronic Allograft Arteriopathy and caTCMR

- Chronic allograft vasculopathy can occur in association with chronic active TCMR, chronic ABMR, or a combination of both.
- In this case, caTCMR was the likely driver, in the absence of DSA or histologic/molecular evidence of antibodies activity.

Understanding caTCMR (Banff 2017 Update)

- Chronic active TCMR was defined in Banff 2017 to include interstitial inflammation in areas of interstitial fibrosis and tubular atrophy (i-IFTA) and was intended to better capture the chronic, active nature of T cell-mediated injury in kidney transplant and to improve the prognostic stratification for graft outcomes [3].
- i-IFTA is strongly associated with graft loss and could reflect an ongoing alloimmune injury, especially in under-immunosuppressed patients or those with prior episodes of acute TCMR [4].
- Importantly, i-IFTA is not specific to rejection—it may also be seen in BK nephropathy, recurrent pyelonephritis, and chronic ABMR.

Prognosis and Treatment Response

- Prognosis for caTCMR is poor across most studies.
- Only about 20% of patients show meaningful improvement in graft function following intensified immunosuppressive therapy [5].
- Early identification and management remain critical, though durable responses are limited.

Rationale for Belatacept Conversion

- In selective stable or low immunologic risk patients with progressive chronic allograft changes or Recipients with vascular lesions (Banff cv Score > 2) switching from CNI to belatacept is associated with improved or stabilized eGFR, reduced development of de novo donor-specific antibodies (dnDSA), and superior long-term graft survival compared to continued CNI therapy [6, 7].

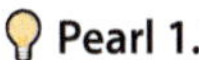

Pearl 1.2

This case highlights the subtle yet progressive nature of chronic T cell-mediated rejection and underscores the importance of molecular diagnostics, biopsy interpretation, and careful immunosuppression adjustment in long-term transplant care.

Case 1.3

Case Study Summary

Patient: A 43-year-old female with end-stage renal disease (ESRD) of unknown etiology.

Transplant course: She underwent a second kidney transplant from an unrelated living donor. Her immunological profile was notable for highly sensitized status due to repeated transplant with a calculated panel-reactive antibody (cPRA) of 54%. She received induction treatment with ATG and steroids, followed by tacrolimus, mycophenolate mofetil (MMF) combination, and daily prednisone; she was later switched to azathioprine due to gastrointestinal intolerance to MMF.

Post-transplant Clinical Course: Subsequent increase in donor-derived cell-free DNA (dd-cfDNA) levels led to a diagnostic biopsy, revealing borderline histological changes. A second biopsy approximately 1-year post-transplant indicated significant fibrosis and chronic active T cell-mediated rejection (TCMR) features.

Diagnosis

- Chronic active T cell-mediated rejection (caTCMR); inflammation in areas of interstitial fibrosis and tubular atrophy (i-IFTA) based on pathologic diagnosis (Figs. 1.6 and 1.7).

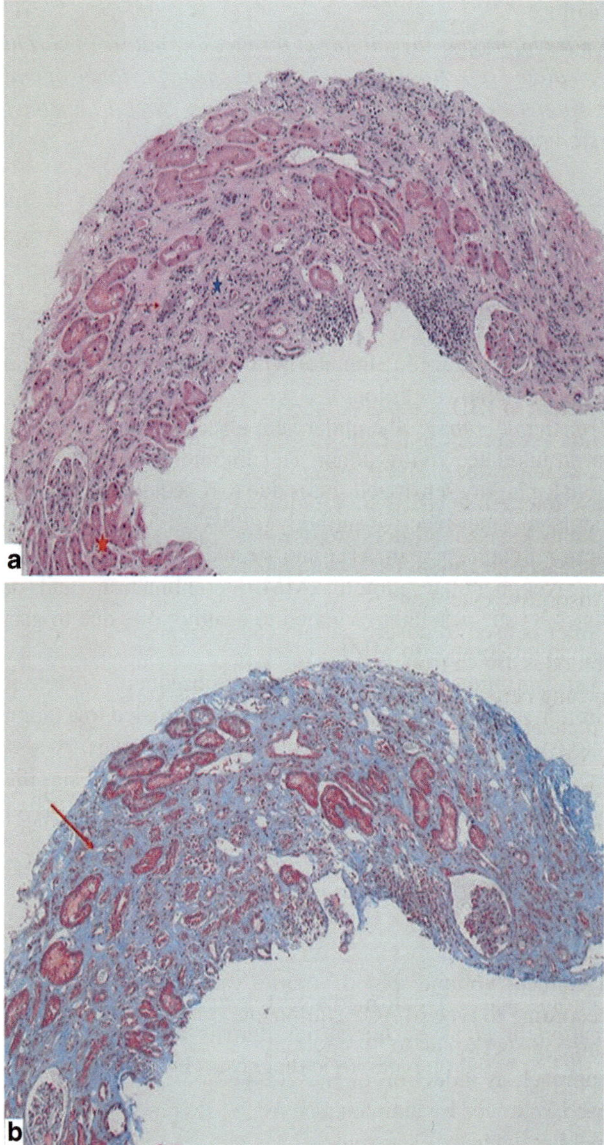

Fig. 1.6 (**a**) iIFTA (blue star) with inflammation, interstitial fibrosis, tubular atrophy, and lymphocytic tubulitis (red arrow) compared with normal-looking uninvolved renal cortex (red star). H&E stain, 10×. (**b**) Interstitial fibrosis (blue stain of the increased interstitial collagen), red arrow. Trichrome stain, 10×

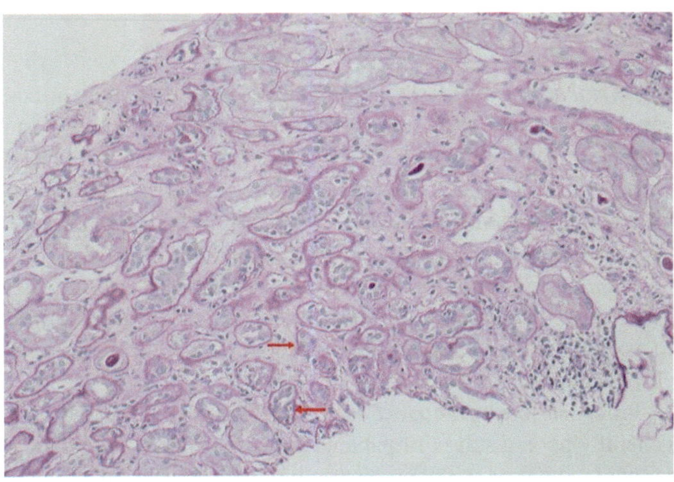

Fig. 1.7 Higher magnification highlighting atrophic cortical tubules (red arrows). PAS, 20×

Management Strategy

Potential contributing factor: Underimmunosuppression and non compliance to medications may have played a role in the development of caTCMR.

Treatment: Immunosuppressive adjustments: Administered corticosteroids to abate ongoing tissue inflammation. Switched from azathioprine back to MMF, increased tacrolimus trough level goals.

Case Follow-Up

- The patient exhibited a slow decline in graft function over the following 5 years.
- Referred for a third kidney transplant assessment.

Educational Insights

Understanding CA TCMR: Chronic active TCMR is an identified variant of kidney allograft rejection associated with long-term graft loss [3].

Diagnostic Criteria: Diagnosis requires the presence of tubulointerstitial inflammation with a score > 2 in both atrophic and non-atrophic areas, as per the Banff 2019 classification [8].

Etiology: Chronic active T cell-mediated rejection (caTCMR) is strongly associated with underimmunosuppression in kidney transplant recipients, particularly in those with progressive chronic allograft changes [9].

Prognosis and Treatment Response: While the prognosis is generally poor, a subset of patients may experience improvement in kidney function with appropriate immunosuppressive therapy.

Pearl 1.3

This case underscores the importance of vigilant monitoring and individualized immunosuppressive therapy in kidney transplant recipients to prevent and manage chronic active TCMR.

Case 1.4

Case Study Summary

Patient: A 23-year-old female with end-stage renal disease (ESRD) of unknown etiology.

Transplant course: She underwent a living unrelated kidney transplant (LUKT) with a poorly matched human leukocyte antigen (HLA) profile. She was highly sensitized with a calculated panel-reactive antibody (cPRA) of 50%.

Post-transplant Clinical course: Traditional induction with ATG and steroids, followed by tacrolimus and azathioprine, mycophenolate mofetil (MMF) was discontinued due to gastrointestinal intolerance.

Six months after transplant and during a routine follow-up, an increase in donor-derived cell-free DNA (dd-cfDNA) was noted and prompted a diagnostic kidney biopsy that confirmed antibody-mediated rejection (ABMR). She received comprehensive treatment including plasmapheresis (PLEX), intravenous immunoglobulin (IVIG), and her immunosuppression was adjusted by reintroducing MMF.

Approximately 2 years post-transplant, a second biopsy revealed severe interstitial fibrosis and tubular atrophy (IFTA) accompanied by features of iIFTA.

Diagnosis

- Main pathological features were interstitial fibrosis and tubular atrophy with inflammation (i-IFTA) (Figs. 1.8 and 1.9).
- Chronic active T cell-mediated rejection (caTCMR) likely related to allograft injury from previous ABMR, underimmunosuppression, or ongoing active rejection.

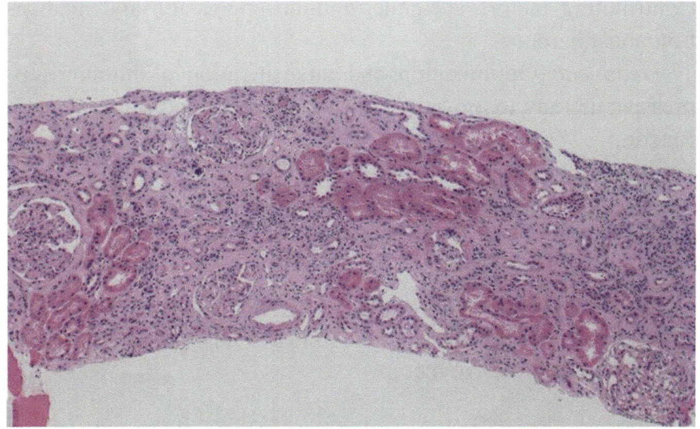

Fig. 1.8 iIFTA with inflammation and tubulitis. H&E, 10×

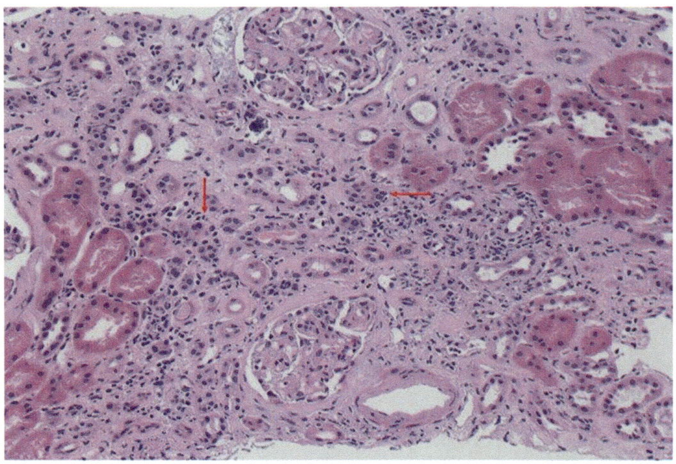

Fig. 1.9 Higher view of iIFTA with inflammation and tubulitis, red arrows. H&E, 20×

Treatment Approach

Contributing factors are underimmunosuppression and medication nonadherence.

Treatment: Optimization and intensification of immunosuppressive therapy to prevent further graft injury and preserve graft function.

Follow-Up

- The patient has maintained stable graft function 4 years after transplantation (latest clinic visit), supported by ongoing immunosuppressive therapy.

Educational Insights

Pathophysiological Uncertainty: The exact mechanistic relationship between i-IFTA and chronic rejection remains unclear. It is debated whether i-IFTA directly contributes to chronic rejection or represents a nonspecific marker of allograft injury like in this case.

Association with Immunosuppression: Clinical studies have demonstrated that i-IFTA often correlates with underimmunosuppression and is frequently preceded by episodes of acute TCMR. This suggests that patients presenting with i-IFTA may benefit from enhanced immunosuppressive therapy [4, 10].

Potential Risks of Overtreatment: Conversely, if i-IFTA simply reflects irreversible tissue injury rather than active rejection or underimmunosuppression, aggressive treatments such as steroids and anti–T-cell therapies may constitute overtreatment and should be carefully considered.

Pearl 1.4

This case highlights the complexities in managing chronic allograft injury, emphasizing the importance of careful interpretation of biopsy findings such as iIFTA and tailored immunosuppression to balance the risks of rejection and overtreatment.

Case 1.5

Case Study Summary

Patient: A 57-year-old male with end-stage renal disease (ESRD) secondary to IgA nephropathy.

Transplant course: Immunologically he was not sensitized; he underwent a living unrelated kidney transplant (LUKT) from a wife. Induction with ATG and steroids, maintenance medications included tacrolimus, prednisone, and mycophenolate.

Post-transplant Clinical course:

Approximately 1 month after transplantation, his creatinine nadir remain elevated for which he had a diagnostic kidney biopsy that revealed significant interstitial fibrosis (IFTA), this was thought to be in relation to calcineurin inhibitor (CNI) toxicity.

- Three months after transplant patient was transitioned to belatacept as a rescue treatment. Tacrolimus was rapidly tapered; this was complicated by the development of oliguric acute kidney injury (AKI) with serum creatinine up to 10 mg/dL.
- Notably, there were no donor-specific antibodies (DSA), and donor-derived cell-free DNA (dd-cfDNA) was only slightly elevated at 0.3%.

Diagnosis

- Grade 3 T cell-mediated rejection (TCMR) with vasculitis features (Banff V3) (Fig. 1.11).
- Evidence of fibrin thrombi and parenchymal infarction with hemorrhage (Figs. 1.10 and 1.11).

Management Approach

Risk factors: Rapid withdrawal of CNI during transition to belatacept early on after transplant.

Treatment:

- Administered intravenous methylprednisolone.
- Received ATG (thymoglobulin) for 8 days.
- One-time dose of eculizumab.
- Resumption of calcineurin inhibitor (CNI) therapy.

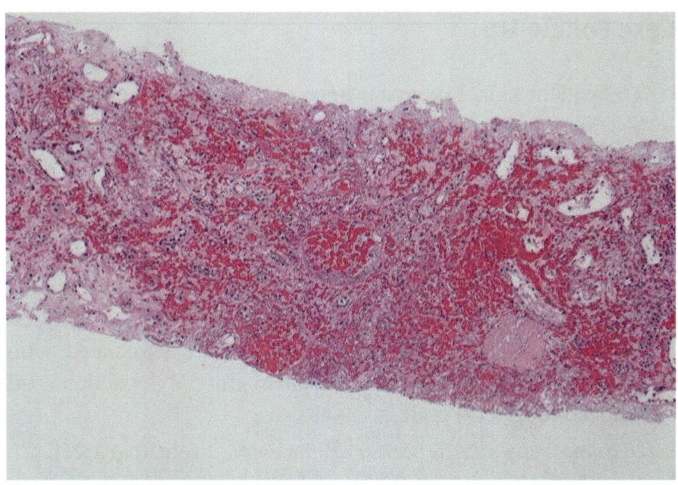

Fig. 1.10 Coagulative necrosis and hemorrhage consistent with parenchymal infarction. H&E, 10×

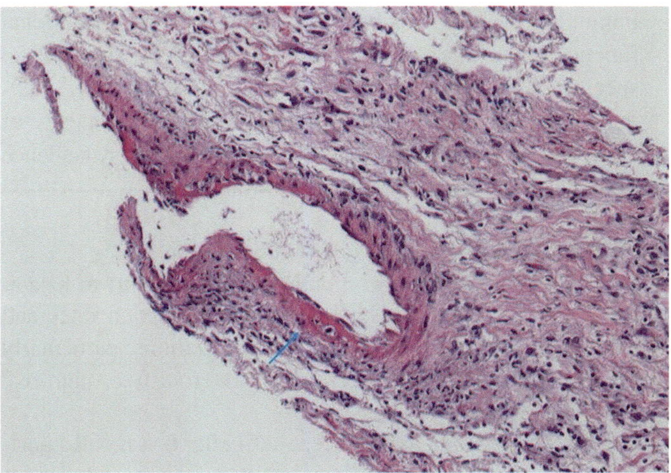

Fig. 1.11 Arterial wall fibrinoid necrosis and transmural inflammation (blue arrow), v3 arteritis. H&E, 20×

Case Follow-Up

- The patient kidney function improved and maintained a stable baseline around 3 years after transplantation date (the latest clinic visit), with a diagnosis of chronic kidney disease stage 3b.

Educational Insights

- *Calcineurin Inhibitor Nephrotoxicity:* CNIs are integral to post-transplant immunosuppression but are associated with nephrotoxicity, leading to chronic graft dysfunction and reduced long-term graft survival.
- *Belatacept as an Alternative*: Belatacept, a selective T cell co-stimulation blocker, is approved for the prophylaxis of kidney transplant rejection.
- *Outcomes of CNI to Belatacept Conversion:* Switching stable renal transplant recipients from CNI-based to belatacept-based immunosuppression has been associated with improved renal function and a similar rate of death or graft loss. However, in specific cases such as in rapid CNI taper or early post-transplant conversion it may lead to a higher incidence of biopsy-proven acute rejection (BPAR) and a lower incidence of de novo donor-specific antibodies (dnDSA) [7].

Timing of Conversion

Early conversion (within 3–6 months post-transplant) to belatacept has been associated with higher acute rejection rates and increased rates of infection-related hospitalizations, particularly cytomegalovirus (CMV) infections in steroid-free high-risk groups [11–13].

Delaying conversion to belatacept until after 6–8 months post-transplant may reduce the risk of acute rejection and serious infections.

Pearl 1.5

This case underscores the complexities in managing kidney transplant recipients, particularly regarding the timing and approach to immunosuppressive therapy. It highlights the importance of balancing the risks of nephrotoxicity with the potential for acute rejection when considering transitions in immunosuppressive regimens.

Case 1.6

Case Study Summary

Patient: A 38-year-old male with end-stage renal disease (ESRD) secondary to granulomatosis with polyangiitis (GPA).

Transplant course: He underwent a deceased donor kidney transplant (DDKT). He had a calculated panel-reactive antibody (cPRA) of 0%. Induction therapy included antithymocyte globulin (ATG), steroids, followed by maintenance triple immunosuppression.

Post-transplant Clinical course:

The post-transplant course was complicated by a low-grade BK viremia, prompting a reduction in Mycophenolate mofetil. Subsequently, tacrolimus was discontinued by hematology-oncology due to a new diagnosis of large granular lymphocytic leukemia (LGL), confounded to be related to post-transplant lymphoproliferative disorder (PTLD). Tacrolimus was replaced by everolimus.

The patient later developed progressive allograft dysfunction with a serum creatinine increase to 6.7 mg/dL. Kidney allograft biopsy revealed severe T cell-mediated rejection (TCMR), confirmed by both histopathology and Molecular Microscope Diagnostic (MMDx). De novo class II donor-specific antibodies (DSAs) were detected (total MFI about 30,000). Antinuclear antibodies (ANA) were positive with a speckled pattern at 1:160. Complement levels and hepatitis serologies were within normal limits, and EBV PCR was undetectable.

Diagnosis

- Severe T Cell-Mediated Rejection (TCMR grade III)—confirmed by biopsy and MMDx diagnostics platform (Fig. 1.12).
- De novo class II DSA.
- Large granular lymphocytic (LGL) leukemia.

Management Approach

Triggering factors: iatrogenic under-immunosuppression.

Treatment:

- High-dose corticosteroids.
- Antithymocyte globulin (ATG).
- Reinstating tacrolimus and mycophenolate mofetil-based therapy.

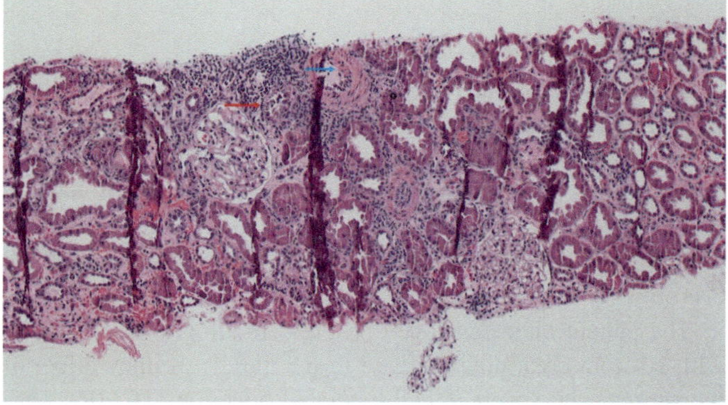

Fig. 1.12 Interstitial inflammation, tubulitis (red arrow), and vasculitis (endotheliitis with fibrinoid necrosis). H&E, 10×

Case Follow-Up

Despite aggressive anti-rejection therapy, the patient's graft function continued to deteriorate. Ultimately, he experienced graft failure and returned to dialysis.

Educational Points

TCMR III

- TCMR III represents the most severe form of cellular rejection and is a strong independent predictor of graft loss.

Large Granular Lymphocytic (LGL) Leukemia

- A clonal lymphoproliferative disorder characterized by splenomegaly and cytopenias.
- Pathogenesis may be genetic or driven by chronic antigen stimulation.
- Commonly associated with autoimmune diseases (e.g., rheumatoid arthritis) [14].
- Must be differentiated from EBV-driven PTLD, which presents with distinct pathology and therapeutic implications.

Management of LGL Versus PTLD

- LGL leukemia often follows an indolent course. Treatment is typically conservative (observation), unless associated with cytopenias, splenomegaly, or autoimmune manifestations, in which case immunosuppressive therapy is indicated.
- PTLD, particularly B-cell type and EBV-positive, has a different approach, starting by reducing immunosuppression and selectively initiating targeted therapies (e.g., rituximab).

 **Pearl 1.6**

This case highlights the importance of correctly distinguishing LGL leukemia from PTLD. Misguided reduction of immunosuppression led to severe rejection and graft loss, emphasizing the need for accurate diagnosis and tailored immunosuppressive management in transplant patients.

Case 1.7

Case Study Summary

Patient: A 41-year-old female with end-stage renal disease (ESRD) due to rapidly progressive glomerulonephritis (RPGN) of unknown etiology. She had previously experienced graft failure after a first living kidney transplant (LKT).

Transplant Course: A second LKT was performed; her cPRA was 54%. Induction therapy included antithymocyte globulin (ATG) and steroids, followed by triple maintenance immunosuppression based on tacrolimus and MMF.

Post-ttransplant Clinical course:

- Mycophenolate mofetil (MMF) was discontinued early due to gastrointestinal intolerance and replaced with azathioprine.
- At 18 months post-transplant, serum creatinine increased from baseline (1.0 mg/dL) to 1.5 mg/dL. Donor-specific antibodies (DSA) remained undetectable; however, donor-derived cell-free DNA (dd-cfDNA) climbed significantly from 0.2% to 1.0%.

Diagnosis

- Chronic active T cell-mediated rejection (CA-TCMR) with severe interstitial fibrosis and tubular atrophy (IFTA) confirmed on biopsy (Figs. 1.13 and 1.14).

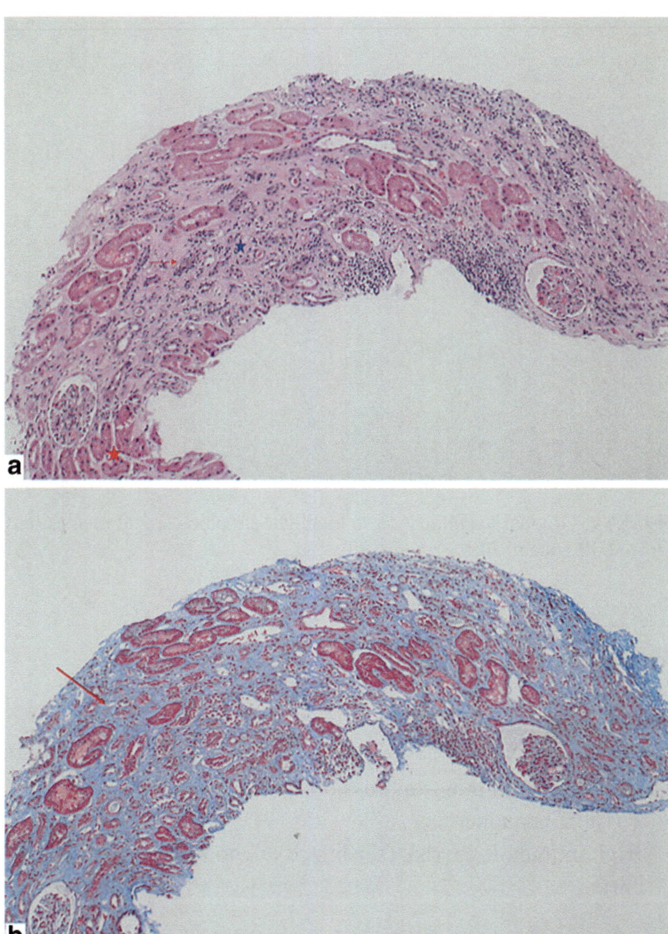

Fig. 1.13 (**a**) iIFTA (blue star) with inflammation, interstitial fibrosis, tubular atrophy, and lymphocytic tubulitis (red arrow) compared with normal looking uninvolved renal cortex (red star). H&E, 10×. (**b**) Interstitial fibrosis (blue stain of the increased interstitial collagen), red arrow. Trichrome stain, 10×

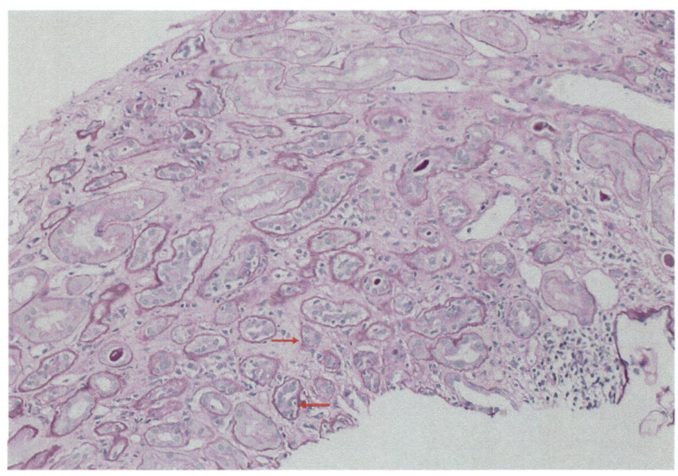

Fig. 1.14 Original magnification to highlight atrophic cortical tubules (red arrows). PAS stain, 20×

Management Approach

Contributing factors:

- Suboptimal immunosuppression.
- Possible nonadherence.
- High immunologic risk (sensitized due to re-transplant recipient).

Treatment:

- Steroids, reintroduction of MMF, and targeting higher levels of tacrolimus.
- Second round of intravenous corticosteroids and antithymocyte globulin (ATG).

Follow-Up

- At 5 years post-transplant, the patient's graft function progressed to stage 4 chronic kidney disease (CKD).
- Repeat biopsy pathology was notable for caTCMR with significant i-IFTA and chronic allograft injury.

Educational Insights

Chronic Active T Cell-Mediated Rejection (CA-TCMR)

A well-defined subtype of rejection characterized histologically by inflammation within areas of interstitial fibrosis and tubular atrophy (i-IFTA), which may signal ongoing alloimmune injury even in the absence of DSA.

Prognosis and Treatment

CA-TCMR is associated with poor response to therapy and long-term graft dysfunction. The role of intensified immunosuppression remains uncertain, and histologic markers (e.g., t score, ci + ct, i score) do not consistently predict treatment response [9, 15].

Monitoring Tools:

- dd-cfDNA can serve as an early non-invasive marker of allograft injury, particularly useful when DSA is absent.
- In the context of CA-TCMR, dd-cfDNA is frequently elevated, though typically to a lesser degree than in ABMR, and can identify ongoing alloimmune injury before changes in serum creatinine or overt graft dysfunction occur [16, 17].

Pearl 1.7

This case underscores the diagnostic and therapeutic challenges of chronic active T cell-mediated rejection (CA-TCMR), particularly in highly sensitized patients. It highlights the importance of maintaining adequate immunosuppression and monitoring biomarkers like dd-cfDNA, as CA-TCMR often presents without DSA and is associated with poor treatment response and progressive graft dysfunction.

References

1. Aubert O, et al. Cell-free DNA for the detection of kidney allograft rejection. Nat Med. 2024;30:2320–7.
2. Bu L, et al. Clinical outcomes from the assessing donor-derived cell-free DNA monitoring insights of kidney allografts with longitudinal surveillance (ADMIRAL) study. Kidney Int. 2022;101(4):793–803.
3. Haas M, et al. The Banff 2017 kidney meeting report: revised diagnostic criteria for chronic active T cell-mediated rejection, antibody-mediated rejection, and prospects for integrative endpoints for next-generation clinical trials. Am J Transplant. 2018;18(2):293–307. https://doi.org/10.1111/ajt.14625.
4. Nankivell BJ. The causes, significance and consequences of inflammatory fibrosis in kidney transplantation: the Banff I-Ifta lesion. Am J Transplant. 2018;18(2):364–76. https://doi.org/10.1111/ajt.14609.
5. Kung VL, Sandhu R, Haas M, Huang E. Chronic active T cell–mediated rejection is variably responsive to immunosuppressive therapy. Kidney Int. 2021;100(2):391–400.
6. Gupta G. Safe conversion from tacrolimus to Belatacept in high immunologic risk kidney transplant recipients with allograft dysfunction. Am J Transplant. 2015;15(10):2726–31. https://doi.org/10.1111/ajt.13322.
7. Bertrand D, et al. Belatacept rescue conversion in kidney transplant recipients with vascular lesions (Banff cv score >2): a retrospective cohort study. Nephrol Dial Transplant. 2023;38(2):481–90. https://doi.org/10.1093/ndt/gfac178.
8. Loupy A. The Banff 2019 kidney meeting report (I): updates on and clarification of criteria for T cell- and antibody-mediated rejection. Am J Transplant. 2020;20(9):2318–31. https://doi.org/10.1111/ajt.15898.
9. Nakagawa K. Significance of revised criteria for chronic active T cell-mediated rejection in the 2017 Banff classification: surveillance by 1-year protocol biopsies for kidney transplantation. Am J Transplant. 2021;21(1):174–85. https://doi.org/10.1111/ajt.16093.
10. Lefaucheur CT. Cell-mediated rejection is a major determinant of inflammation in scarred areas in kidney allografts. Am J Transplant. 2018;18(2):377–90. https://doi.org/10.1111/ajt.14565.

11. Tawhari I. Early Calcineurin-inhibitor to Belatacept conversion in steroid-free kidney transplant recipients. Front Immunol. 2022;13:1096881. https://doi.org/10.3389/fimmu.2022.1096881.
12. Chavarot N. Increased incidence and unusual presentations of CMV disease in kidney transplant recipients after conversion to Belatacept. Am J Transplant. 2021;21(7):2448–58. https://doi.org/10.1111/ajt.16430.
13. Noble J, Leon J. Belatacept in kidney transplantation: reflecting on the past, shaping the future. Transpl Int. 2025;38:14412. https://doi.org/10.3389/ti.2025.14412.
14. Marchand T. Large granular lymphocyte leukemia: a clonal disorder with autoimmune manifestations. Hematol Am Soc. 2024;2024(1):143–9. https://doi.org/10.1182/hematology.2024000539.
15. Kung VL. Chronic active T cell-mediated rejection is variably responsive to immunosuppressive therapy. Kidney Int. 2021;100(2):391–400. https://doi.org/10.1016/j.kint.2021.03.027.
16. Gauthier PT. Distinct molecular processes mediate donor-derived cell-free DNA release from kidney transplants in different disease states. Transplantation. 2024;108(4):898–910. https://doi.org/10.1097/TP.0000000000004877.
17. Bloom RD. Cell-free DNA and active rejection in kidney allografts. J Am Soc Nephrol. 2017;28(7):2221–32. https://doi.org/10.1681/ASN.2016091034.

Alloimmune Kidney Injury: Antibodies Mediated Rejection (AMR)

2

Hasan Fattah

Case 2.1

Case Study Summary

Patient: A 63-year-old male past medical history for end-stage renal disease (ESRD) secondary to autosomal dominant polycystic kidney disease (ADPKD).

Transplant History: Second kidney transplant from living unrelated donor (LUKT), 4/6 human leukocyte antigen (HLA) mismatch, highly sensitized.

Post-transplant Clinical course:

- Post-transplant baseline creatinine 1.2 mg/dl.
- He was switched from tacrolimus (due to side effects) to cyclosporine, target cyclosporine trough: 100–150 ng/mL, MMF 1000 mg BID, prednisone 5 mg daily.
- Routine follow-up and labs at 6 months post-transplant: at baseline creatinine, trace proteinuria on the urinalysis; however, donor-derived cell-free DNA (dd-cfDNA) was elevated at

H. Fattah (✉)
Jacob School of Medicine and Biomedical Science, University at Buffalo, Buffalo, NY, USA

H. Fattah, V. Cornea (eds.), *Transplantation in Practice*,
https://doi.org/10.1007/978-3-032-15908-3_2

6% (baseline normal range < 1%), with emerging de novo donor-specific antibodies (DSAs). Total MFI 14,000 (against multiple donor specific antigens).

Diagnosis

Histology: Active antibody-mediated rejection (aABMR) with evidence of microvascular inflammation (MVI) (Figs. 2.1 and 2.2).

Molecular Diagnostics: Severe ABMR signature based on molecular transcriptomes.

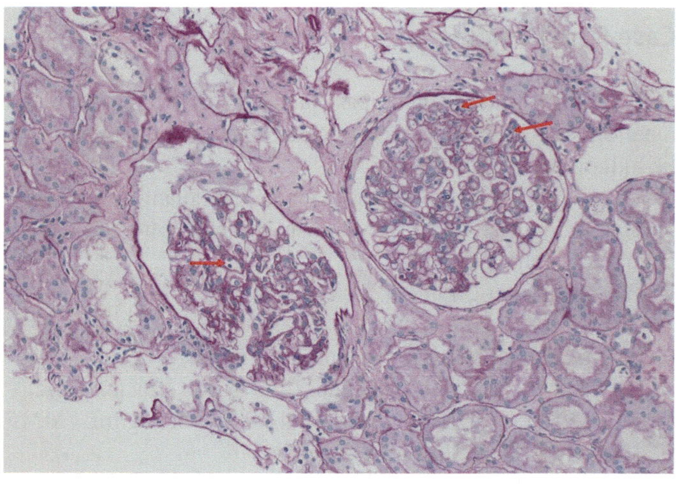

Fig. 2.1 Glomerulitis (g, intracapillary leukocytes). PAS stain, 20×

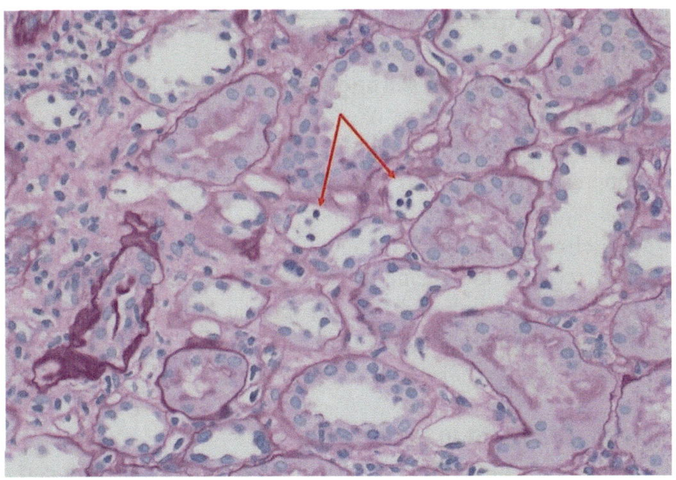

Fig. 2.2 Peritubular capillaritis (PTC, red arrows). PAS stain, 20×

Treatment Approach

- Therapeutic plasma exchange (TPE) combined with Intravenous immunoglobulin (IVIG).
- Pulse corticosteroids.
- Conversion from cyclosporine to tacrolimus.
- Course of bortezomib.

Case Follow-Up

- Creatinine, remained stable; proteinuria, increased; and ARBs were added.
- dd-cfDNA: Down to 2.6% remained elevated but stable throughout the most recent clinic visit.
- DSA: significant reduction of total antibodies to 2500 MFI total.

Educational Insights

Immunosuppression Management in High-Risk Recipients

- It may be ideal to maintain maximally tolerated triple immunosuppression in high-risk transplant group.
- The Kidney Disease Improving Global Outcomes (KDIGO) guideline [1] and several meta-analyses report that tacrolimus reduces the incidence of acute rejection by approximately 12% compared to cyclosporine during the first-year post-transplant, with rates such as 22% vs. 42% at 12 months in some studies [2].

Role of dd-cfDNA in Monitoring

- Donor-derived cell-free DNA could serve as a sensitive early marker for graft injury and rejection.
- It can be detected up to 5 months before biopsy-proven antibody-mediated rejection and 2 months before T cell-mediated rejection, whereas serum creatinine lacks this early discriminatory power [3].

Chronic Active ABMR (caABMR)

- Early detection and preemptive management are key to preserving long-term graft function.
- Early post-transplant modification in immunosuppressive strategy (e.g., switching to cyclosporine) should be carefully evaluated in high-risk patients (Figs. 2.3 and 2.4).

Pearl 2.1

This case emphasizes the critical need for vigilant monitoring and tailored immunosuppression strategies in high-risk transplant recipients. It also showcases the value of integrating molecular diagnostics and noninvasive biomarkers into clinical practice.

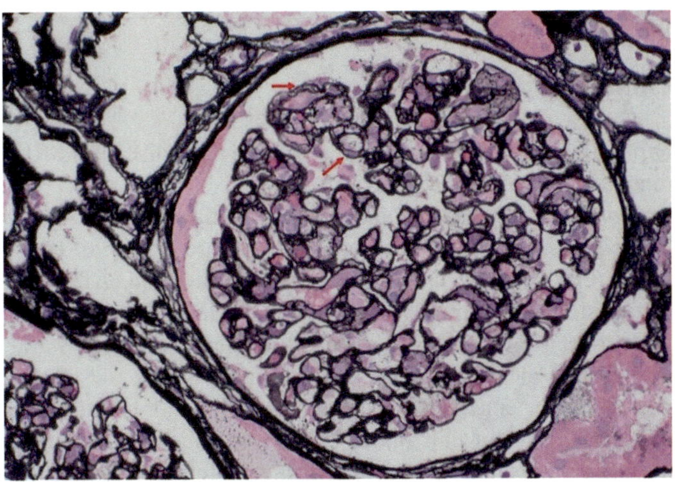

Fig. 2.3 Original magnification to show cg (double contours of GBM, "tram track," red arrows). Silver Jones stain, 40×

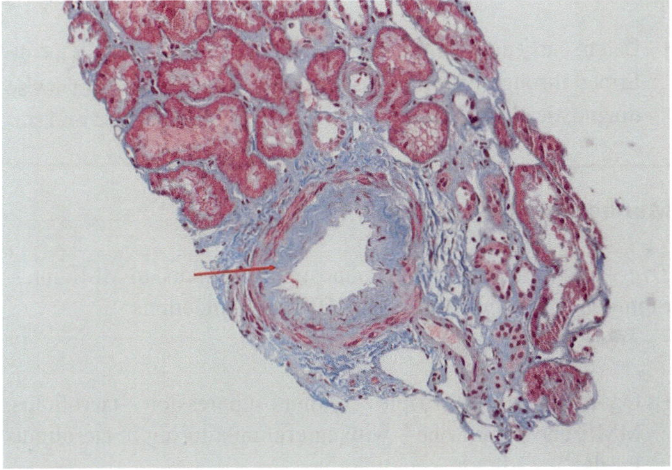

Fig. 2.4 Arterial fibroelastosis (fibrointimal thickening, red arrow). Trichrome stain, 20×

Case 2.2

Clinical Study Summary

Patient: A 48-year-old male with end-stage renal disease (ESRD) secondary to IgA nephropathy.

Transplant course: He underwent a living unrelated kidney transplant (LUKT). He was non-sensitized at the time of transplant (cPRA 0%). Induction treatment included ATG and Corticosteroids, followed by tacrolimus, MMF, and prednisone.

Post-transplant Clinical course: Routine surveillance works up revealed elevated donor-derived cell-free DNA (dd-cfDNA >60%) and the emergence of de novo class II donor-specific antibodies (DSA) following a brief COVID-19 infection and temporary discontinuation of mycophenolate mofetil (MMF) due to gastrointestinal side effects.

Diagnosis

- Latent early active antibody-mediated rejection (ABMR), confirmed through histologic assessment (Fig. 2.5) and molecular diagnostics MMDx.

Management Approach

Triggering Factor: Under-immunosuppression due to MMF interruption and possible impact of COVID-19 infection.

Treatment:

- Optimization of triple immunosuppression—tacrolimus, MMF, and prednisone—with careful monitoring of tacrolimus levels.

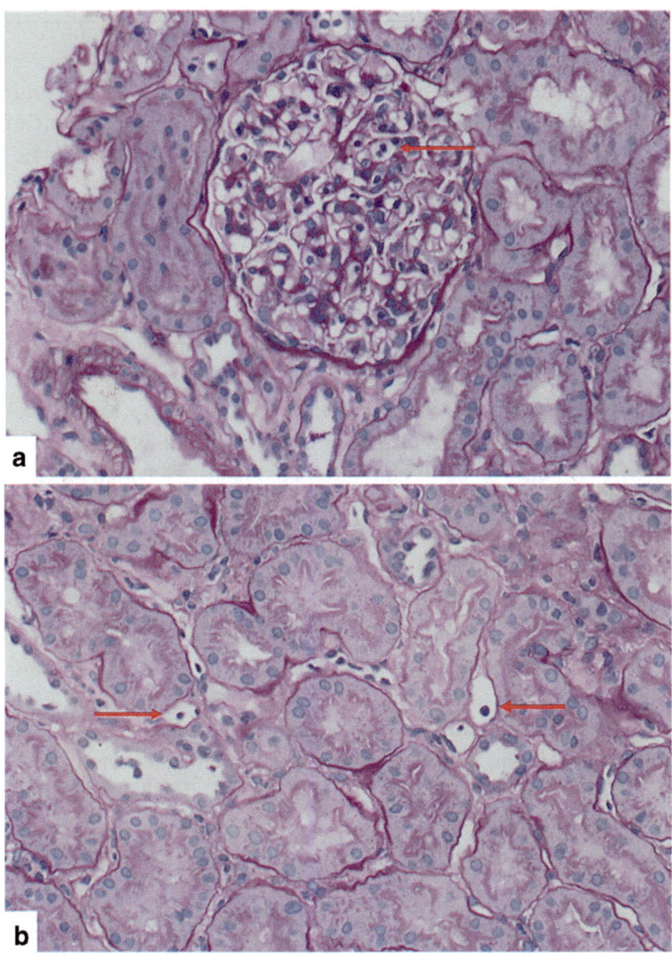

Fig. 2.5 (**a**) Glomerular intracapillary lymphocytes consistent with glomerulitis, red arrow. PAS, 40×. (**b**) peritubular capillaries with intralumenal lymphocytes consistent with peritubular capillaritis, red arrows. PAS, 40×

Case Follow-Up

- At 3 years post-transplant, the patient maintained stable graft function with resolution of DSA, highlighting the benefit of early intervention and close monitoring in subclinical ABMR.

Educational Insights

- Subclinical ABMR is frequently encountered and should not be considered a benign entity, as it may progress silently and impact long-term graft survival.
- Early diagnosis through detection of noninvasive biomarkers (dd-cfDNA, DSA) and utilizing molecular diagnostics (e.g., MMDx) may be particularly valuable in at-risk patients [4].
- The ideal target tacrolimus trough level during the first year after kidney transplantation is 5–8 ng/mL, with many guidelines and large cohort studies supporting a range of 7–12 ng/mL in the early post-transplant period (first 3–6 months), then 5–8 ng/mL through the remainder of the first year [5, 6]; low levels are associated with increased risk of de novo DSA formation.
- Molecular diagnostics using transcriptomic profiling and machine learning–based algorithms can enhance histopathologic interpretation, improving early rejection detection and guiding treatment decisions [7].

Pearl 2.2

This case highlights the importance of vigilant monitoring for subclinical antibody-mediated rejection, particularly after episodes of under-immunosuppression. Even in non-sensitized patients, events like temporary immunosuppression withdrawal and infections can trigger de novo *DSA formation. Early detection using biomarkers and molecular diagnostics enables timely intervention, which can preserve graft function and improve long-term outcomes.*

Case 2.3

Case Study Summary

Patient: A 62-year-old female with a history of NASH cirrhosis and chronic kidney disease stage 4 (CKD4) secondary to diabetes mellitus.

Transplant course: She underwent a combined liver-kidney transplant (SLK). She was highly sensitized with a cPRA of 81%. Induction treatment with basiliximab and intravenous steroids, maintenance treatment was based on Tacrolimus and prednisone.

Post-transplant clinical course:

- Post-transplant, the patient had chronic severe leukopenia attributed to hypersplenism, which precluded the use of anti-metabolite therapy.
- She subsequently developed chronic active antibody-mediated rejection (ABMR) with nephrotic-range proteinuria. Kidney biopsy confirmed chronic active ABMR and transplant glomerulopathy (Figs. 2.6 and 2.7).

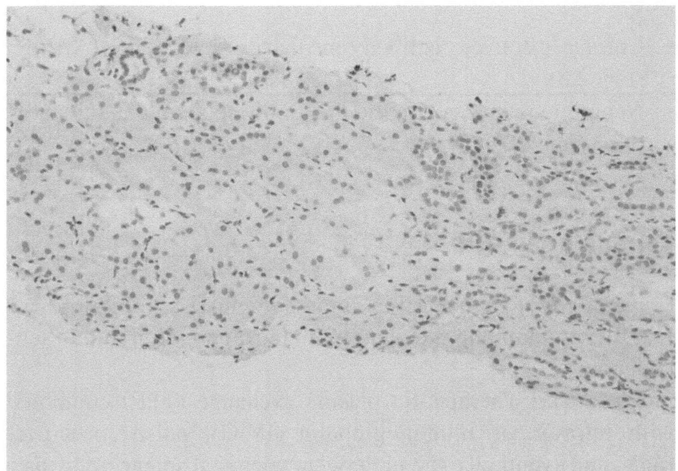

Fig. 2.6 Negative staining for C4d. IHC, 20×

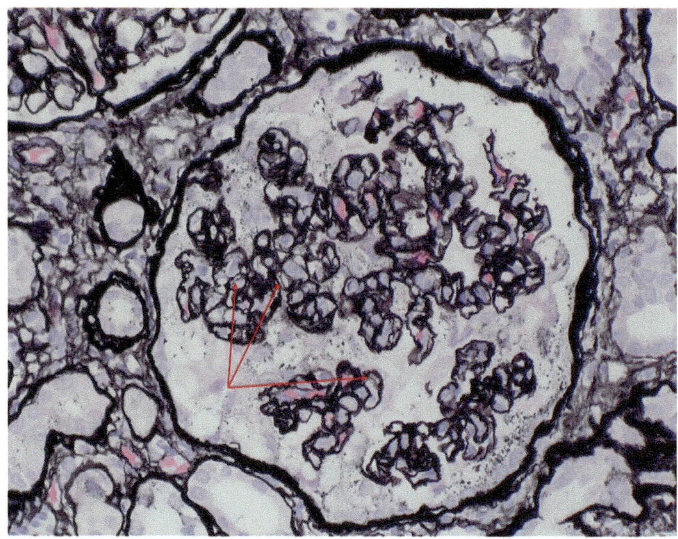

Fig. 2.7 GBM double contours consistent with transplant glomerulopathy (TG), red arrows. Silver Jones stain, 40×

Diagnosis

- Chronic active antibody-mediated rejection (ABMR) (Fig. 2.8).
- Nephrotic range proteinuria due to transplant glomerulopathy (TG) (Fig. 2.7).

Management Approach

Contributing Factors: High immunologic risk (cPRA 81%). Inability to maintain adequate immunosuppression due to leukopenia.

Treatment: Therapeutic plasma exchange (TPE) combined with intravenous immunoglobulin (IVIG), pulse corticosteroids, and eventually she underwent chemical splenectomy as a last resort to reverse leukopenia and to be able to resume antimetabolites.

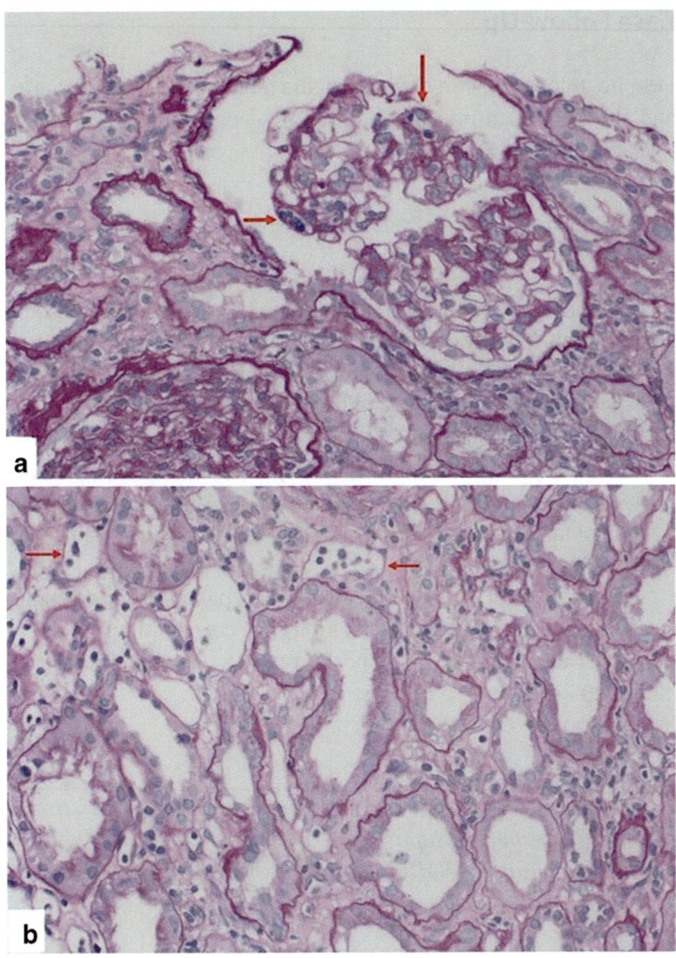

Fig. 2.8 (**a**) glomerulitis (red arrows) PAS, 40× (**b**) Peritubular capillaritis (red arrows). PAS, 40×

Case Follow-Up

Despite treatment, renal function did not recover significantly, and the patient ultimately required a second kidney transplant 2 years after the initial SLK.

Educational Insights

- Combined liver-kidney transplantation is traditionally associated with lower rates of rejection due to the liver's immunomodulatory effects [8]. However, this protection is not absolute or guaranteed particularly in highly sensitized recipients.
- Under-immunosuppression is a well-established risk factor for the development of de novo donor-specific antibodies (dnDSA) and chronic antibody-mediated rejection (AMR) in solid organ transplantation, including simultaneous liver-kidney transplant (SLK) recipients [9].
- Management of ABMR in such complex patients requires individualized approaches, such as surgical correction of underlying causes (e.g., splenectomy) to enable adequate immunosuppressive therapy.

Pearl 2.3

This case highlights that even in combined liver-kidney transplants, under-immunosuppression in highly sensitized patients can lead to chronic ABMR, and graft loss, emphasizing the need to maintain adequate immunosuppression.

Case 2.4

Case Study Summary

Patient: A 51-year-old male with end-stage renal disease (ESRD) of unknown etiology.

Transplant course: He underwent deceased donor kidney transplantation (DDKT); he was not sensitized, panel reactive antibody (cPRA) 0%. He received induction therapy with ATG and steroids and kept on maintenance triple immunosuppression based on tacrolimus and MMF.

Post-transplant Clinical course:

- Eight years post-transplant, the patient presented with a rise in serum creatinine from 1.0 to 1.4 mg/dL, accompanied by moderate proteinuria. Workup revealed de novo donor-specific antibodies (DSAs), primarily against class II. BK virus testing and imaging were unremarkable.
- Allograft biopsy demonstrated features consistent with chronic active antibody-mediated rejection (ABMR), including morphologic changes of transplant glomerulopathy (TG).

Diagnosis

Chronic active ABMR with histologic evidence of transplant glomerulopathy (Figs. 2.9 and 2.10).

Management Approach

Contributing Factors: medication nonadherence, the patient had independently discontinued corticosteroids, raising concerns regarding medication non-adherence as a potential trigger for alloimmune injury.

Treatment: Optimization of immunosuppression and plasmapheresis (PLEX) to mitigate the effects of ongoing alloimmune activity role of PLEX is very limited.

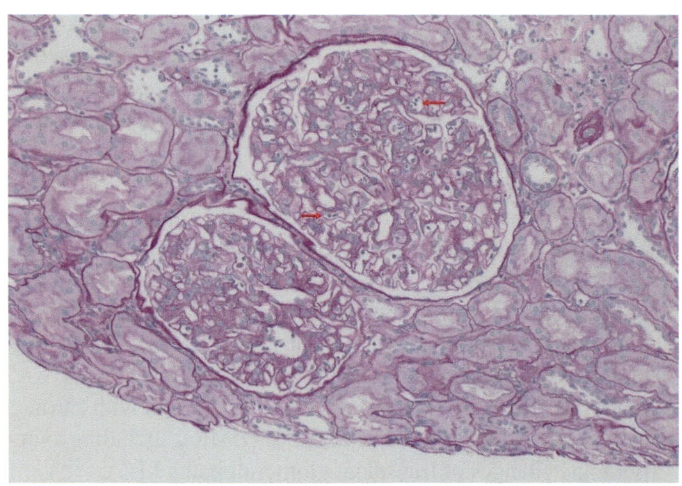

Fig. 2.9 Intracapillary leukocytes (glomerulitis), red arrows. PAS, 20×

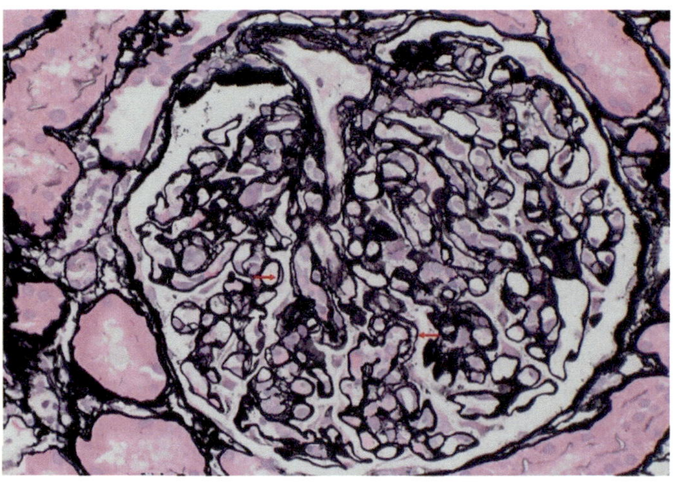

Fig. 2.10 GBM double contours, red arrows. Jones methenamine silver stain, 40×

Case Follow-Up

Unfortunately, the patient succumbed to complications related to COVID-19. Notably, the kidney graft remained functional at the time of death.

Educational Insights

Transplant glomerulopathy (TG) is a non-specific histopathological pattern seen in renal allografts and is not a stand-alone diagnosis. It is characterized by duplication of the glomerular basement membrane (GBM), observable on light or electron microscopy, without immune complex deposition.

Etiology of TG reflects chronic, nonspecific recurrent endothelial injury. Potential mechanisms include [10]:

- Alloimmune injury mediated by HLA donor-specific antibodies (DSAs).
- Autoantibody responses.
- Cell-mediated immune mechanisms.
- Thrombotic microangiopathy.
- Chronic infections such as hepatitis C.

Clinical Presentation: TG can be asymptomatic and detected on protocol biopsy or present with clinical signs such as:

- Proteinuria, potentially reaching the nephrotic range.
- Hypertension.
- Progressive decline in graft function.

Pearl 2.4

The presence of TG is associated with reduced long-term graft survival, emphasizing the importance of early detection and ensuring optimal adherence to immunosuppressive therapy.

Case 2.5

Case Study Summary

Patient: A 45-year-old female with a history of end-stage renal disease (ESRD) secondary to IgA nephropathy.

Transplant course: She underwent living unrelated kidney transplant (LUKT). Induction treatment included ATG and steroids. Current maintenance immunosuppression includes tacrolimus, and mycophenolate mofetil (MMF).

Post-transplant Clinical course:

- The patient presented 7 years after transplant with a rising serum creatinine (from baseline 1.5 mg/dL to 2.0 mg/dL), mild proteinuria (0.4 g/day), and microscopic hematuria. Donor-specific antibodies (DSA) were present with a mean fluorescence intensity (MFI) of 17,000. Donor-derived cell-free DNA (dd-cfDNA) was elevated at 2.5%.
- A renal allograft biopsy revealed histological changes consistent with recurrent IgA nephropathy.
- Electron microscopy demonstrated features suggestive of chronic active antibody-mediated rejection (ABMR), including glomerular capillary double contours and multilayering of peritubular capillary basement membranes.

Diagnosis

- Recurrent IgA nephropathy based on light microscopy (Figs. 2.11 and 2.12).
- Chronic active ABMR and early TG based on EM (Fig. 2.11).

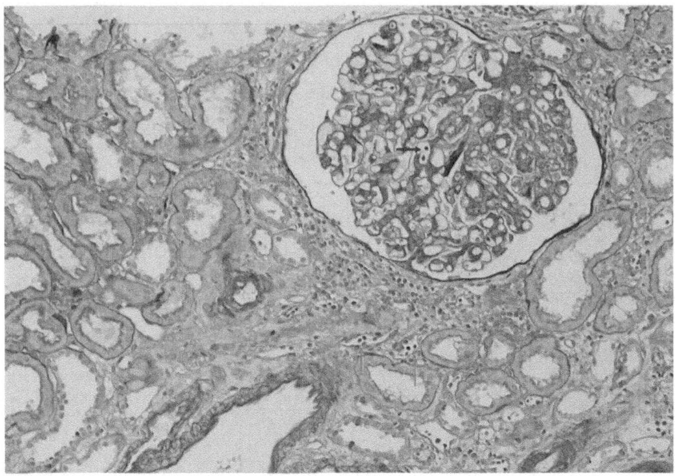

Fig. 2.11 Glomerular intracapillary leukocytes (glomerulitis, red arrow) and peritubular capillaritis (blue arrows). PAS, 20×

Management Approach

Identified Trigger: Under-immunosuppression is the likely the key contributing factor to graft dysfunction and alloimmune activation.

Treatment:

- Initiation of corticosteroid therapy.
- Optimization of immunosuppression regimen.

Case Follow-Up

The patient has maintained stable graft function at 11 years post-transplant (the latest follow-up with transplant clinic).

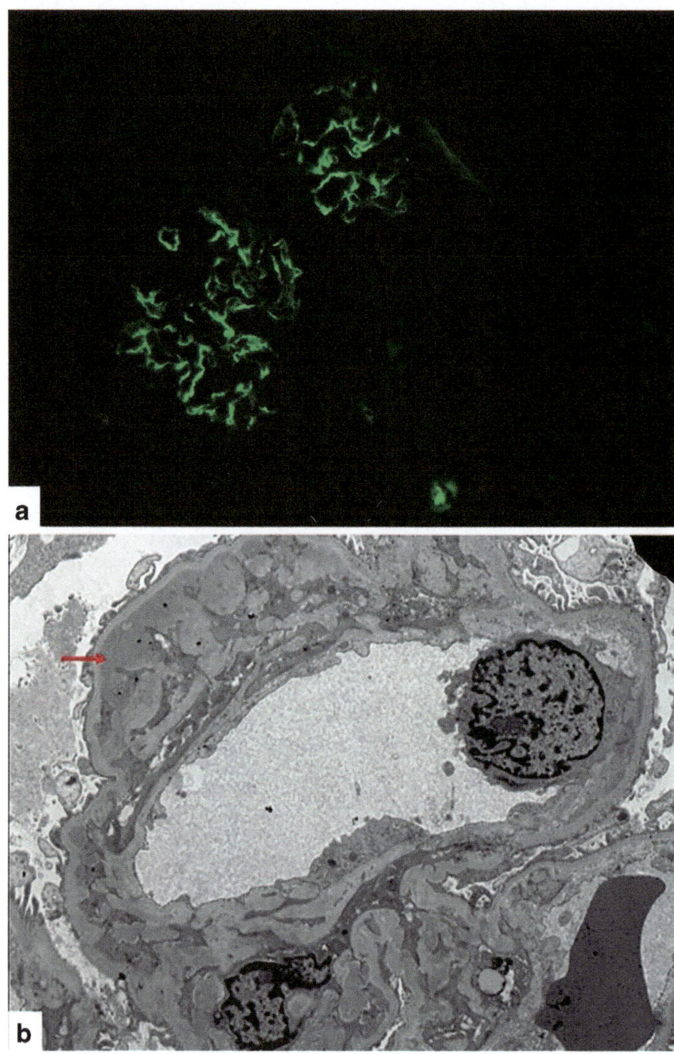

Fig. 2.12 (**a**) mesangial staining IgA immune complex deposits. Immunofluorescence, 20×. (**b**) mesangial electron dense deposits, red arrow. Electron microscopy, 1200×

Educational Insights

Combined Biomarker Utility:

The use of both DSA and dd-cfDNA provides improved sensitivity and specificity for the detection of ABMR compared to either test alone [11, 12].

Recurrence of IgA Nephropathy:

Recurrence is common and often subclinical. Therefore, histological findings should be interpreted cautiously within the clinical context to avoid over- or under-treatment.

Pathology Interpretation Challenges:

Histologic evaluation of microvascular inflammation (MVI) and ABMR is prone to inter-observer variability [13]. A multidisciplinary approach, incorporating serological and molecular diagnostics (e.g., DSA, dd-cfDNA), improves diagnostic accuracy and reduces the risk of missed ABMR.

Pearl 2.5

This case underscores the need for a multimodal approach to graft dysfunction. Recurrent IgA and ABMR can coexist, and combining biopsy with DSA and dd-cfDNA improves diagnostic accuracy. Careful interpretation prevents missed or delayed treatment.

Case 2.6

Cast Study Summary

Patient: 28-year-old female with ESRD secondary to Wilms tumor.

Transplant course: She received a living-related kidney transplant (LRKT). Pre-transplant cPRA was 45%, and immunosuppression included ATG and steroids induction, followed by combination of tacrolimus, prednisone, and everolimus.

Post-transplant Clinical course:

- The patient presented 3 years after transplant with acute kidney injury (creatinine increased from 1.3 mg/dL to 2.4 mg/dL).
- Initial evaluation revealed no detectable donor-specific antibodies (DSA), a negative non-HLA antibody screen (including AT1R and MICA), nonreactive urinary sediment, and normal imaging. Notably, donor-derived cell-free DNA (dd-cfDNA) was elevated at 4.9%.
- Two allograft biopsies showed only nonspecific findings—acute tubular injury and borderline changes.

Diagnosis

- Equivocal nonspecific findings on repeated pathology samples (Fig. 2.13).
- Moderate, fully developed antibody-mediated rejection (ABMR) confirmed via molecular diagnostics (MMDx).

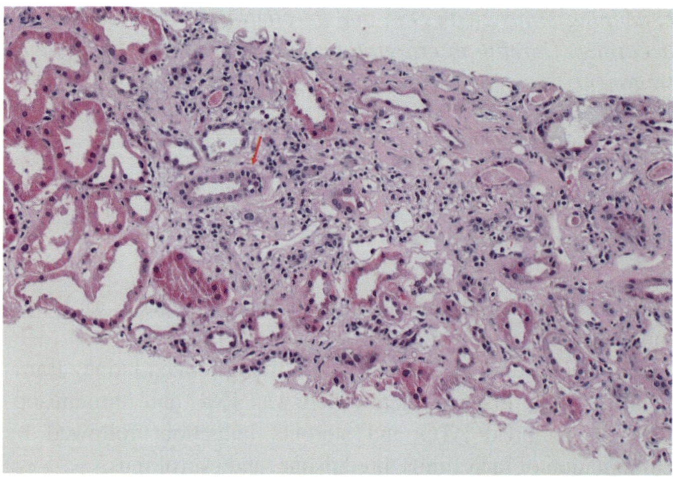

Fig. 2.13 Interstitial inflammation and mild tubulitis (t1), red arrow. Nonspecific changes under microscope that do not meet the Banff criteria for rejection. H&E, 20×

Management Approach

- Discontinuation of everolimus, and initiation of mycophenolate mofetil (MMF).
- Increased tacrolimus trough target level.
- A pulse corticosteroids.
- Conversion to belatacept.

Case Follow-Up

The patient maintains stable allograft function 8 years post-transplant, with new baseline CKD and serum creatinine at 2.0 mg/dL (up to the latest documented clinic visit).

Educational Insights

Limitations of Banff Criteria:

Multiple studies demonstrate that a significant proportion of ABMR cases lack detectable DSA or C4d positivity and that histologic features alone may not capture the full spectrum of ABMR [14].

Role of Molecular Diagnostics:

Molecular platforms such as donor-derived cell free DNA (cfDNA) and MMDx which uses genetic expression analysis can be valuable in specific clinical cases where traditional biopsy findings are inconclusive or does not meet Banff criteria for rejection [15].

Therapeutic Considerations in Late ABMR (after 6 months of transplant):

Optimizing immunosuppression.

Belatacept may be a viable alternative to calcineurin inhibitors (CNIs) in late-stage conversion for kidney transplant recipients experiencing chronic antibody-mediated rejection (ABMR) [16].

 **Pearl 2.6**

This case highlights that antibody-mediated rejection can occur despite negative DSA and inconclusive biopsy findings. Molecular diagnostics like ddcfDNA and MMDx are valuable tools to identify such cases.

Case 2.7

Case Study Summary

Patient: A 33-year-old male with end-stage renal disease (ESRD) secondary to IgA nephropathy.

Transplant course: He underwent deceased donor kidney transplantation (DDKT) with a pre-transplant panel reactive antibody (cPRA) of 0%. Induction with (ATG), steroids, and maintenance triple immunosuppression were initiated.

Post-transplant Clinical course:

Three years after transplant, the patient developed nephrotic-range proteinuria and clinical nephrotic syndrome. Evaluation revealed the emergence of de novo donor-specific antibodies (DSA) and markedly elevated donor-derived cell-free DNA (dd-cfDNA) at 11%.

Allograft biopsy demonstrated recurrent subclinical IgA nephropathy alongside chronic active antibody-mediated rejection (ABMR).

Diagnosis

Chronic active antibody-mediated rejection (Figs. 2.14 and 2.15).

Management Approach

Over the subsequent 5 years, the patient underwent multiple biopsies confirming persistent chronic active ABMR. Treatment regimens included variety of medications including corticosteroids,

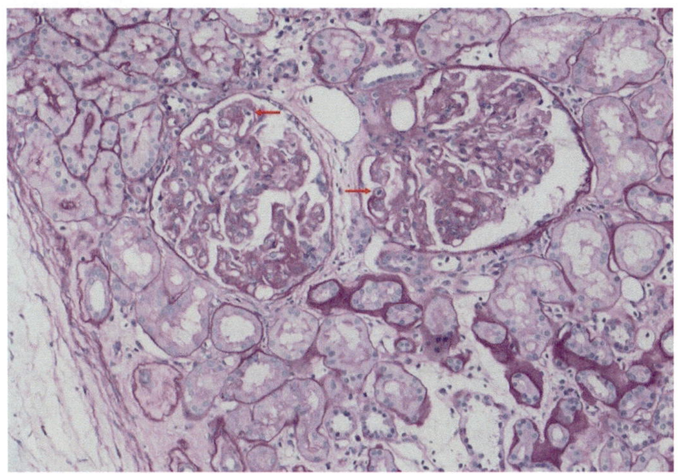

Fig. 2.14 Intracapillary lymphocytes (glomerulitis), red arrow. PAS, 20×

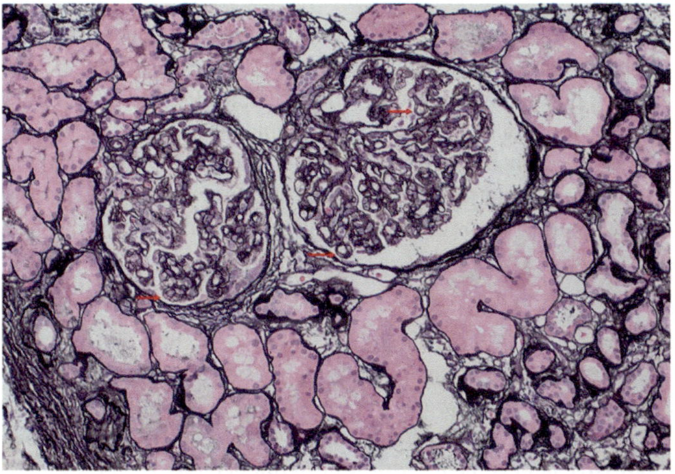

Fig. 2.15 GBM double contours (TG). Methenamine Jones silver stain, 20×

plasmapheresis (PLEX), rituximab, bortezomib, and eventually conversion to Belatacept.

Case Follow-Up

Despite aggressive therapy, the patient continued to have slow but progressive chronic kidney disease to stage 4 around 9 years after kidney transplant (latest visits on records).

Educational Insights

Treatment and clinical presentation challenges:

- Alloimmune injury is typically indolent, progressive, and driven by complex humoral and cellular mechanisms that are not adequately targeted by current immunosuppressive regimens.
- Late chronic active ABMR is difficult to manage and often shows limited response to conventional therapies.
- Such disappointing results reinforce a need of new innovative treatment strategies, and improved understanding of its molecular mechanisms and the definition of diagnostic criteria [17].
- Nephrotic syndrome and heavy proteinuria can be the presenting manifestations of ABMR, underscoring the need for timely evaluation.

Pearl 2.7

This case illustrates the challenging nature of late chronic active ABMR, which often shows poor response to standard therapies. Persistent DSA and elevated dd-cfDNA warrant early biopsy and aggressive management to slow allograft decline.

References

1. Chapman JR. The KDIGO clinical practice guidelines for the care of kidney transplant recipients. Transplantation. 2010;89(6):644–5.
2. Margreiter R. Efficacy and safety of tacrolimus compared with ciclosporin microemulsion in renal transplantation: a randomised multicentre study. Lancet. 2002;359(9308):741–6. https://doi.org/10.1016/S0140-6736(02)07875-3.
3. Bromberg JS, et al. Elevation of donor-derived cell-free DNA before biopsy-proven rejection in kidney transplant. Transplantation. 2024;108(9):1994–2004. https://doi.org/10.1097/TP.0000000000005007.
4. Obrişcă B. Combining donor-derived cell-free DNA and donor specific antibody testing as non-invasive biomarkers for rejection in kidney transplantation. Sci Rep. 2022;12(1):15061. https://doi.org/10.1038/s41598-022-19017-7.
5. Han A. Optimum tacrolimus trough levels for enhanced graft survival and safety in kidney transplantation: a retrospective multicenter real-world evidence study. Int J Surgery (London, England). 2024;110(10):6711–22. https://doi.org/10.1097/JS9.0000000000001800.
6. Yin S. Non-linear relationship between tacrolimus blood concentration and acute rejection after kidney transplantation: a systematic review and dose-response meta-analysis of cohort studies. Curr Pharm Des. 2019;25(21):2394–403. https://doi.org/10.2174/1381612825666190717101941.
7. Halloran PF, et al. The molecular phenotype of kidney transplants. Am J Transplant. 2010;10(10):2215–22.
8. Simpson N. Comparison of renal allograft outcomes in combined liver-kidney transplantation versus subsequent kidney transplantation in liver transplant recipients: analysis of UNOS database. Transplantation. 2006;82(10):1298–303. https://doi.org/10.1097/01.tp.0000241104.58576.e6.
9. O'Leary JG. Class II alloantibody and mortality in simultaneous liver-kidney transplantation. Am J Transplant. 2013;13(4):954–60. https://doi.org/10.1111/ajt.12147.
10. Edward FJ. Transplant glomerulopathy. Mod Pathol. 2018;31(2):235–52. https://doi.org/10.1038/modpathol.2017.123.
11. Halloran PF. Antibody-mediated rejection without detectable donor-specific antibody releases donor-derived cell-free DNA: results from the trifecta study. Transplantation. 2023;107(3):709–19. https://doi.org/10.1097/TP.0000000000004324.
12. Mayer KA. Diagnostic value of donor-derived cell-free DNA to predict antibody-mediated rejection in donor-specific antibody-positive renal allograft recipients. Transplantation. 2021;34(9):1689–702. https://doi.org/10.1111/tri.13970.

13. Delsante M. Microvascular inflammation in renal allograft biopsies assessed by endothelial and leukocyte co-immunostain: a retrospective study on reproducibility and clinical/prognostic correlates. Transpl Int. 2019;32(3):300–12. https://doi.org/10.1111/tri.13371.
14. Halloran PF. Molecular diagnosis of ABMR with or without donor-specific antibody in kidney transplant biopsies: differences in timing and intensity but similar mechanisms and outcomes. Am J Transplant. 2022;22(8):1976–91. https://doi.org/10.1111/ajt.17092.
15. Gupta G. Correlation of donor-derived cell-free DNA with histology and molecular diagnoses of kidney transplant biopsies. Transplantation. 2022;106(5):1061–70. https://doi.org/10.1097/TP.0000000000003838.
16. Kumar D. Impact of Belatacept conversion on renal function, histology, and gene expression in kidney transplant patients with chronic active antibody-mediated rejection. Transplantation. 2021;105(3):660–7. https://doi.org/10.1097/TP.0000000000003278.
17. Böhmig GA. The therapeutic challenge of late antibody-mediated kidney allograft rejection. Transpl Int. 2019;32(8):775–88. https://doi.org/10.1111/tri.13436.

Alloimmune Kidney Injury: Mixed T and B Cell-Mediated Rejection

3

Fawad Shuaib

Case 3.1

Case Study Summary

60-year-old African American female with history of end-stage renal disease (ESRD) of unclear etiology. She underwent 4/6 HLA mismatched deceased donor kidney transplant (DDKT), with a calculated PRA (cPRA) 82%. She received immunosuppression induction with antithymocyte globulin (ATG), and maintenance regimen included tacrolimus, mycophenolate mofetil and daily prednisone.

Post-transplant Clinical Course

- Mycophenolate mofetil dose was reduced 2–3 months after transplant due to gastrointestinal side effects and low-grade BK viremia.

F. Shuaib (✉)
Division of Nephrology, Bone and Mineral Metabolism, University of Kentucky, Lexington, KY, USA
e-mail: Fnu.Fawad@uky.edu

H. Fattah, V. Cornea (eds.), *Transplantation in Practice*,
https://doi.org/10.1007/978-3-032-15908-3_3

- 5 months after transplant, her donor-derived cell-free DNA (dd-cfDNA) increased from 0.5% to 2.5%. Additionally, de novo donor-specific antibodies (DSAs) were detected against class 2 HLA antigens. Renal allograft biopsy was performed.

Diagnosis

- Borderline changes of T cell-mediated rejection (TCMR) based on histological examination. No histological features of antibody-mediated rejection (ABMR). See (Figs. 3.1 and 3.2) for mild interstitial inflammation and tubulitis.
- Moderate early-stage antibody-mediated rejection (ABMR) based on molecular biopsy assessment (MMDx). No T cell-mediated rejection (TCMR) on MMDx.

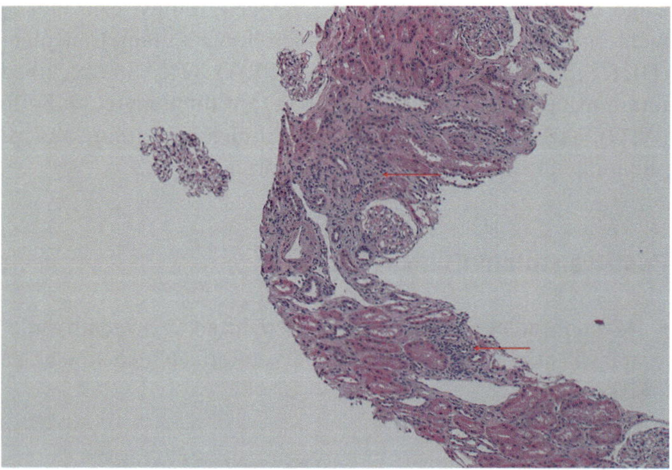

Fig. 3.1 Mild interstitial inflammation (red arrows), H&E, 10×

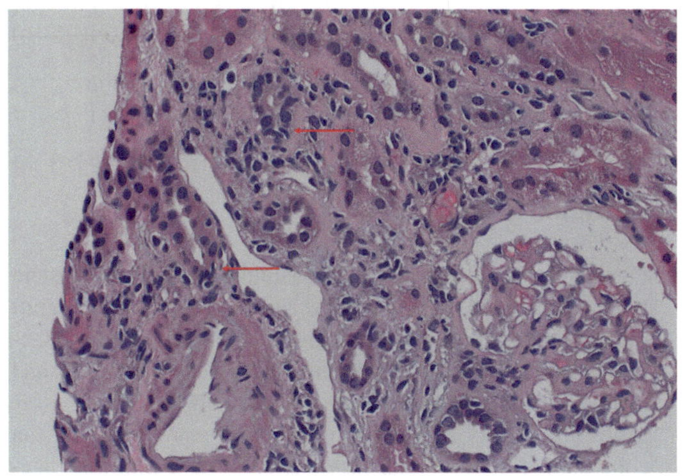

Fig. 3.2 Mild tubulitis (t1) [red arrows]. H&E, 40×

Management Approach

Factors which likely contributed to development of rejection:

- Sensitization (high calculated PRA).
- HLA mismatch.
- Reduction in immunosuppression (mycophenolate mofetil dose was decreased due to gastrointestinal side effects and BK viremia).

Treatment

Steroids and maximization of maintenance immunosuppression regimen.

Follow-Up

- Resolution of DSA and return of dd-cfDNA to baseline.
- Stable graft function at 1 year.

Educational Insight

- Histopathology based diagnosis using Banff scoring system remains the gold standard for diagnosis of kidney allograft rejection, but it has some limitations. The lesions that characterize rejection can also be seen in other disease processes, and there can be significant inter-observer variability [1].
- Molecular biopsy assessment using gene expression data can complement conventional histopathology and improve diagnostic accuracy of allograft rejection [1–3].
- Studies have suggested disagreement between histopathology diagnosis and molecular biopsy assessment in up to 20–37% of the cases [1, 4].
- In cases where such discrepancy exists, results should be interpreted in the context of clinical history, risk factors for alloimmunization, immunosuppression drug levels and noninvasive biomarkers.

Pearl 3.1

This case underscores the limitations of conventional microscopy in diagnosis of rejection. Molecular microscopy augments conventional microscopy and can improve diagnostic accuracy of rejection.

Case 3.2

Case Study Summary

31-year-old white male with history of end-stage renal disease (ESRD) due to congenital anomalies of the kidney and urinary tract (CAKUT). He received 6/6 HLA mismatched living unrelated donor kidney transplant. His calculated PRA was 0%. He received immunosuppression induction with antithymocyte globulin (ATG) and maintenance regimen included tacrolimus, mycophenolate mofetil, and daily prednisone.

Post-transplant Clinical Course

- He developed BK viremia 2 months after kidney transplant which prompted reduction in immunosuppression.
- At around 3 months post-transplant, he was noted to have elevated donor-derived cell-free DNA (dd-cfDNA) up to 2.8% and de novo donor-specific antibodies (DSAs).
- No significant rise in serum creatinine or development of proteinuria was noted. Renal allograft biopsy was performed.

Diagnosis

- Light microscopy showed severe lymphoplasmacytic proliferation (Figs. 3.3 and 3.4) suspicions for post-transplant lymphoproliferative disorder (PTLD).
- Hematopathology evaluation was performed, and it did not show any evidence of involvement by a lymphoproliferative disorder. EBV PCR was not detected in blood.
- A final presumptive diagnosis of acute T-cell mediated rejection (TCMR) Banff grade 1B and equivocal findings of antibody-mediated rejection (ABMR) was made.
- Molecular biopsy assessment was consistent with mild T cell-mediated rejection (TCMR) and moderate early-stage antibody-mediated rejection (ABMR).

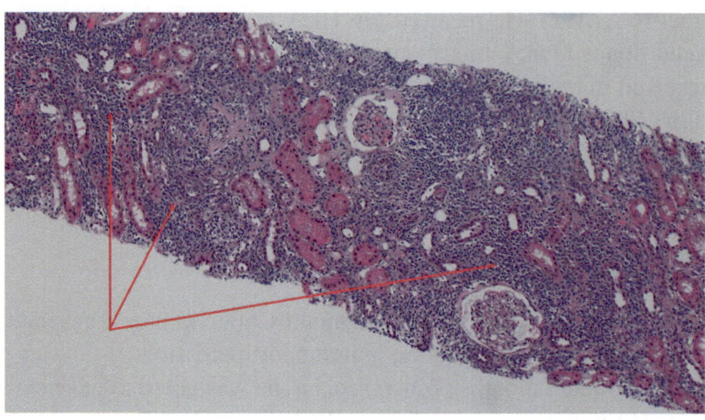

Fig. 3.3 Interstitial lymphoplasmacytic infiltrate, low magnification (red arrows). H&E, 10×

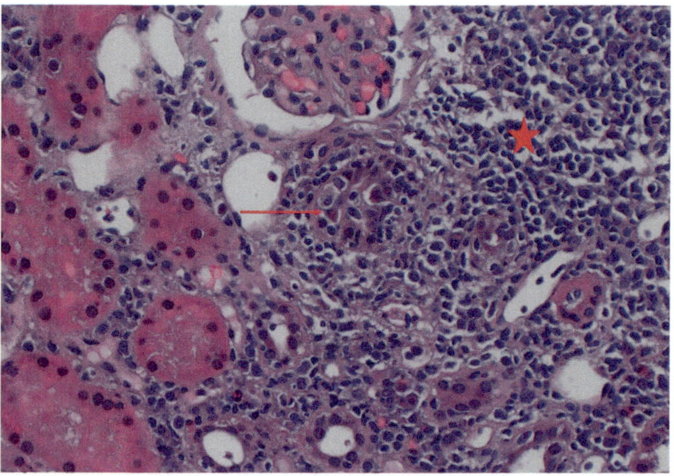

Fig. 3.4 Interstitial inflammation, high magnification (red star) and lymphocytic tubulitis (red arrow). H&E, 40×

Management Approach

- Intravenous steroid pulse.
- Antithymocyte globulin (ATG).
- Plasmapheresis, total of six sessions followed by intravenous immunoglobulin (IVIG).

Follow-Up

- Good response to treatment. Stable allograft function at 1 year.

Educational Insights

- Post-transplant lymphoproliferative disorder (PTLD) is a known complication following kidney transplantation and around one-third to one-half of the cases may involve the renal allograft [5, 6].
- Epstein-Barr virus (EBV) infection and the overall intensity of immunosuppression are known risk factors for PTLD [5].
- Distinguishing between acute rejection and PTLD is important because each entity requires a different treatment approach.
- Severe lymphoplasmacytic proliferation can be seen in both acute rejection and PTLD. Further investigation including hematopathology markers, EBV serology, and molecular tests should be utilized to narrow down the diagnosis [7–9].

Pearl 3.2

This case highlights the histological overlap between some cases of severe acute rejection and PTLD and underscores the importance of other diagnostic tests including, hematopathology, EBV serology and molecular tests to establish the diagnosis.

Case 3.3

Case Study Summary

38-year-old male with end-stage renal disease (ESRD) secondary to polycystic kidney disease. He underwent deceased donor kidney transplant (DDKT). He received immunosuppression induction with antithymocyte globulin (ATG), and maintenance regimen included tacrolimus, mycophenolate mofetil, and daily prednisone.

Post-transplant Clinical Course

- He developed BK viremia early in the course of transplant. He also had diarrhea which was attributed to mycophenolate mofetil (MMF). MMF was discontinued and he was started on everolimus. He was continued on tacrolimus and prednisone.
- Around 5 years after transplant, serum creatinine increased from baseline of 1.3 mg/dL to 1.7 mg/dL. Work up revealed elevated donor-derived cell-free DNA (dd-cfDNA) at 6% and rising donor-specific antibodies to HLA class II antigens. Renal allograft biopsy was performed.

Diagnosis

- Biopsy revealed acute T-cell mediated rejection (TCMR) Banff grade IIA and active antibody-mediated rejection (ABMR) (Figs. 3.5 and 3.6).
- Molecular biopsy assessment (MMDx) confirmed mixed rejection.

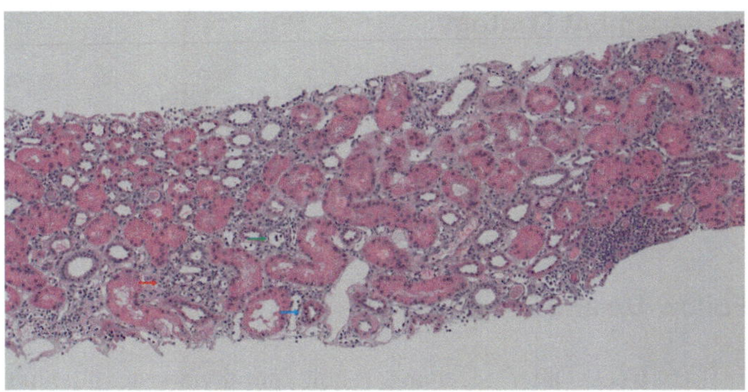

Fig. 3.5 Interstitial inflammation (red arrow), tubulitis (blue arrow) and peritubular capillaritis (green arrow). H&E, 10×

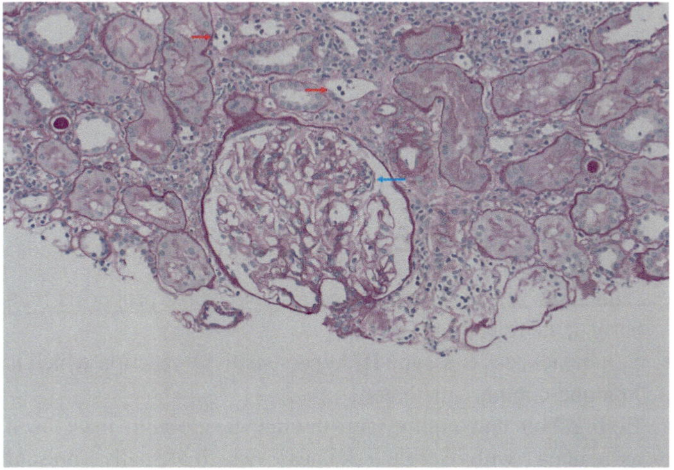

Fig. 3.6 Glomerulitis (blue arrow) and peritubular capillaritis (red arrows). PAS, 20×

Management Strategy

- Rabbit antithymocyte globulin (rATG) and steroids.
- Maximization of maintenance immunosuppression.
- After completion of ATG, also underwent six sessions of plasmapheresis and IVIG.

Follow-Up and Prognosis

- Two weeks after receiving rabbit anti-thymocyte globulin (rATG), he presented with pain in multiple joints and skin rash which was thought to be consistent with serum sickness (Type III hypersensitivity reaction).
- After completion of treatment there was resolution of DSAs, reduction in dd-cfDNA from 6% to 1.1%, and renal allograft function remains stable at 8 years post-transplant.

Educational Insights

- Acute rejection can happen late in the post-transplant course and is usually a consequence of inadequate immunosuppression or noncompliance [10, 11].
- Late acute rejection is believed to have worse prognosis than early acute rejection [10, 11].
- Serum sickness is a Type III hypersensitivity reaction which is immune-complex-mediated.
- Both rabbit and equine anti-thymocyte globulin have been associated with serum sickness which usually present 1–3 weeks after exposure [12, 13].
- Symptoms of serum sickness may include fever, rash, lymphadenopathy, arthralgias, and jaw pain [12, 13].
- Treatment of serum sickness due to anti-thymocyte globulin includes steroids and plasmapheresis in resistant cases [12, 13].

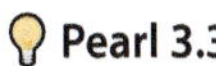

Pearl 3.3

Late acute rejection is usually a consequence of under-immunosuppression or noncompliance. Serum sickness, a Type III immune complex-mediated hypersensitivity reaction can occur after treatment with anti-thymocyte globulin (ATG).

Case 3.4

Case Study Summary

- 29-year-old female with end-stage renal disease (ESRD) secondary to diabetic nephropathy in the setting of Type 1 diabetes mellitus. She underwent living unrelated donor kidney transplant (LUKT). She was not sensitized with calculated PRA of 0%. She received induction with antithymocyte globulin (ATG), and maintenance regimen included tacrolimus, mycophenolate mofetil and prednisone.

Post-transplant Clinical Course

- She had persistent leukopenia which required significant dose reduction of mycophenolate mofetil.
- Ten months post-transplant, she was noted to have new onset proteinuria, rising donor-derived cell-free DNA (dd-cfDNA) to 5.6% from 0.4% previously, and de novo donor-specific antibodies (DSAs) to class 1 and class 2 antigens. Her serum creatinine was unchanged. Renal allograft biopsy was performed.

Diagnosis

- T-cell mediated rejection (TCMR) 1A and chronic active antibody-mediated rejection (ABMR) (Figs. 3.7 and 3.8).

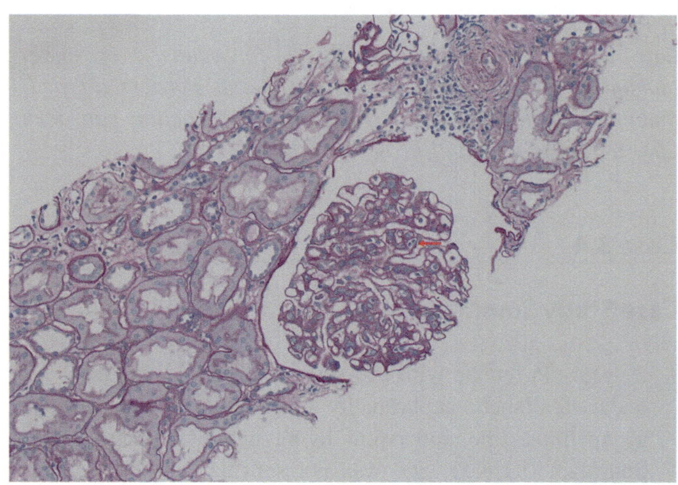

Fig. 3.7 Glomerulitis (red arrow). H&E, 10×

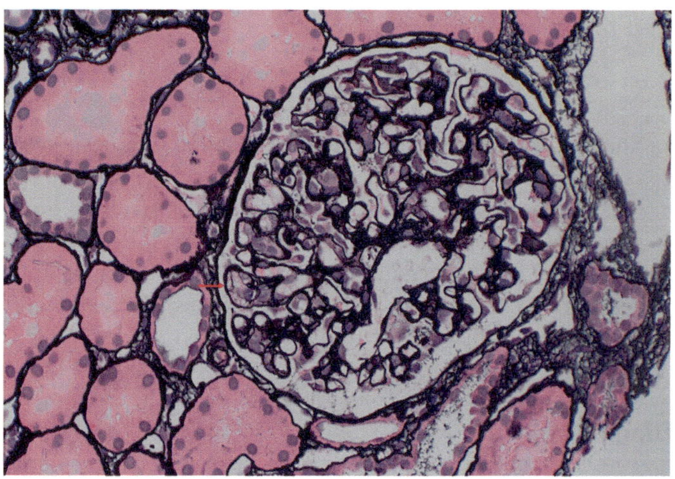

Fig. 3.8 Transplant glomerulopathy (red arrow). Jones methenamine silver stain, 20×

Treatment Approach

- Mixed rejection was treated with steroids, plasmapheresis (PLEX), intravenous immunoglobulin (IVIG), and later required a course of bortezomib due to persistent active rejection.
- She received another cycle of bortezomib and was later transitioned from tacrolimus to belatacept.

Follow-Up

- A repeat biopsy after treatment showed persistent chronic active antibody-mediated rejection (ABMR) with no evidence of significant T cell-mediated rejection (TCMR).
- Despite the evidence of persistent chronic antibody-mediated rejection (ABMR), and the need for further immunosuppression, renal allograft function remains relatively stable at 5 years post-transplant with minimal proteinuria and estimated GFR unchanged from baseline.

Educational Insights

- Mixed rejection of renal allograft is often triggered by under-immunosuppression or medication nonadherence.
- Elevation of serum creatinine level is not a reliable marker of renal allograft rejection as it has limited sensitivity and specificity [14, 15].
- Rise in serum creatinine may be seen relatively late in the course of rejection when significant alloimmune injury has already taken place [14].
- A combination of blood and urine tests should be used to monitor graft health, including monitoring for proteinuria [15].
- Donor-derived cell-free DNA (dd-cfDNA) is a noninvasive biomarker which can be used to monitor for alloimmune injury, and it has the ability to detect subclinical rejection [14, 16, 17].

 **Pearl 3.4**

Serum creatinine can be a lagging marker of renal allograft rejection. Monitoring donor-derived cell-free DNA can allow clinicians to detect alloimmune injury early before it becomes clinically evident.

Case 3.5

Case Study Summary

- 30-year-old female with end-stage renal disease (ESRD) secondary to diabetic nephropathy in the setting of Type 1 diabetes mellitus. She underwent living related kidney transplant (LRKT) from her mother which was a haplotype match. She was not sensitized with calculated PRA of 0%.
- She received immunosuppression induction with basiliximab (Simulect), and maintenance regimen included tacrolimus, mycophenolate mofetil, and prednisone.

Post-transplant Clinical Course

- Serum creatinine started rising in the immediate post-transplant period after an initial mild decline. Urine output also dropped, and patient required three dialysis sessions for volume overload.
- No donor-specific antibodies were detected against the mismatched HLA antigens.
- Endothelial cell crossmatch was positive against EC1 and EC2.
- Renal allograft biopsy was performed on post-operative day 4.

Diagnosis

- Severe acute T cell-mediated rejection (TCMR) Banff grade III (Figs. 3.9 and 3.10) and active antibody mediated rejection (ABMR).

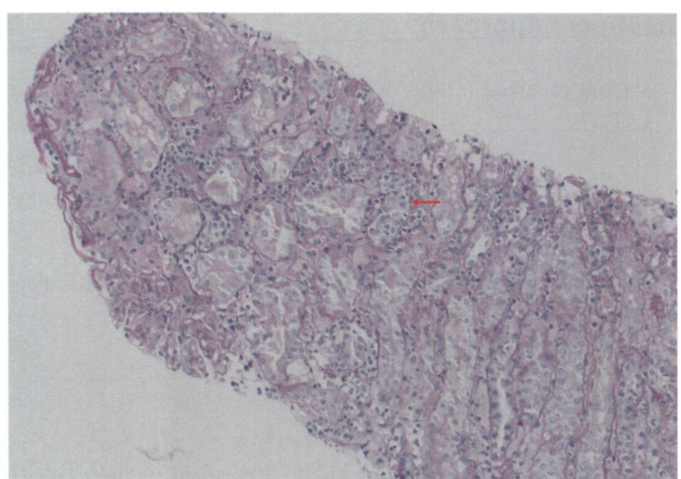

Fig. 3.9 Interstitial inflammation and tubilitis (red arrow). PAS, 20×

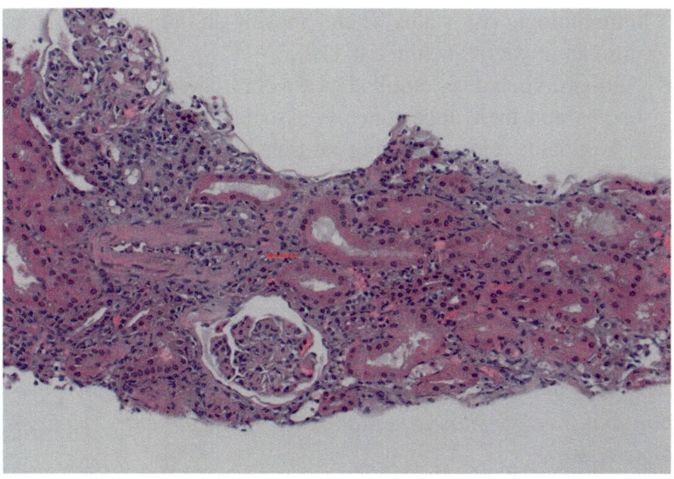

Fig. 3.10 Interstitial inflammation and transmural arteritis (v3) [red arrow]. H&E, 20×

Treatment Approach

- Patient received a total of 7 days of anti-thymocyte globulin (ATG).

Follow-Up

- Excellent response to rejection treatment. Renal allograft function remains stable at 5 years post-transplant.

Educational Insights

- Induction therapies used for kidney transplant include T-cell-depleting agents (antithymocyte globulin) and non-T cell-depleting agents (basiliximab).
- Careful consideration should be given to the patient's overall immunologic risk status when choosing an induction agent as this can impact rejection risk [18].
- Anti-endothelial cell antibodies are considered non-HLA antibodies and their appearance is associated with an increased risk of acute rejection early post-transplantation [19, 20].
- It is not entirely clear if there is a causal relationship between de novo anti-endothelial cell antibodies and rejection or if they simply appear after rejection as a marker of endothelial damage [21].

Pearl 3.5

Induction immunosuppression decreases the risk of acute rejection and therapy should be tailored to each patient's immunologic risk.

Note: This chapter was authored by Dr. Fawad Shuaib. It has been reviewed and edited by Dr. Hasan Fattah, the principal author, to maintain consistency with the rest of the book.

References

1. Reeve J, Einecke G, Mengel M, Sis B, Kayser N, Kaplan B, Halloran PF. Diagnosing rejection in renal transplants: a comparison of molecular- and histopathology-based approaches. Am J Transplant. 2009;9(8):1802–10. https://doi.org/10.1111/j.1600-6143.2009.02694.x.
2. Halloran PF, Reeve J, Akalin E, Aubert O, Bohmig GA, Brennan D, Bromberg J, Einecke G, Eskandary F, Gosset C, Duong Van Huyen JP, Gupta G, Lefaucheur C, Malone A, Mannon RB, Seron D, Sellares J, Weir M, Loupy A. Real time central assessment of kidney transplant indication biopsies by microarrays: the INTERCOMEX study. Am J Transplant. 2017;17(11):2851–62. https://doi.org/10.1111/ajt.14329.
3. Kumar D, Raju N, Tanriover B, Azzouz L, Moinuddin I, Philogene M, Kamal L, McDougan F, Massey HD, Muthusamy S, Lee I, Halloran P, Gupta G. Tissue-based gene expression diagnosis of mild and moderate T-cell-mediated rejection to guide therapy in kidney transplants. Transplantation. 2024; https://doi.org/10.1097/TP.0000000000005296.
4. Madill-Thomsen K, Perkowska-Ptasińska A, Böhmig GA, Eskandary F, Einecke G, Gupta G, Halloran PF. Discrepancy analysis comparing molecular and histology diagnoses in kidney transplant biopsies. Am J Transplant. 2020;20(5):1341–50. https://doi.org/10.1111/ajt.15752.
5. Sprangers B, Riella LV, Dierickx D. Posttransplant lymphoproliferative disorder following kidney transplantation: a review. Am J Kidney Dis. 2021;78(2):272–81. https://doi.org/10.1053/j.ajkd.2021.01.015.
6. Randhawa PS, Magnone M, Jordan M, Shapiro R, Demetris AJ, Nalesnik M. Renal allograft involvement by Epstein-Barr virus associated post-transplant lymphoproliferative disease. Am J Surg Pathol. 1996;20(5):563–71. https://doi.org/10.1097/00000478-199605000-00003.
7. Troxell ML, Dunlap JB, Mittalhenkle A, Ishag M, Fan G, Huang JZ, Gatter K, Byrd DM, Webster D, Houghton DC. Rejection versus post-transplantation lymphoproliferative disorder in a renal transplant recipient. Am J Kidney Dis. 2008;52(6):1174–9. https://doi.org/10.1053/j.ajkd.2008.04.033.
8. Randhawa P, Demetris AJ, Pietrzak B, Nalesnik M. Histopathology of renal posttransplant lymphoproliferation: comparison with rejection using the Banff schema. Am J Kidney Dis. 1996;28(4):578–84. https://doi.org/10.1016/s0272-6386(96)90470-9.
9. Trpkov K, Marcussen N, Rayner D, Lam G, Solez K. Kidney allograft with a lymphocytic infiltrate: acute rejection, posttransplantation lymphoproliferative disorder, neither, or both entities? Am J Kidney Dis. 1997;30(3):449–54. https://doi.org/10.1016/s0272-6386(97)90295-x.

10. Nair R, Agrawal N, Lebaeau M, Tuteja S, Chandran PK, Suneja M. Late acute kidney transplant rejection: clinicopathological correlates and response to corticosteroid therapy. Transplant Proc. 2009;41(10):4150–3. https://doi.org/10.1016/j.transproceed.2009.09.074.
11. Dörje C, Midtvedt K, Holdaas H, Naper C, Strøm EH, Øyen O, Leivestad T, Aronsen T, Jenssen T, Flaa-Johnsen L, Lindahl JP, Hartmann A, Reisæter AV. Early versus late acute antibody-mediated rejection in renal transplant recipients. Transplantation. 2013;96(1):79–84. https://doi.org/10.1097/TP.0b013e31829434d4.
12. Teng J, Hoo XN, Tan SJ, Dwyer K. Serum sickness following rabbit anti-thymocyte globulin for acute vascular renal allograft rejection. Clin Kidney J. 2012;5(4):334–5. https://doi.org/10.1093/ckj/sfs061.
13. Boothpur R, Hardinger KL, Skelton RM, Lluka B, Koch MJ, Miller BW, Desai NM, Brennan DC. Serum sickness after treatment with rabbit anti-thymocyte globulin in kidney transplant recipients with previous rabbit exposure. Am J Kidney Dis. 2010;55(1):141–3. https://doi.org/10.1053/j.ajkd.2009.06.017.
14. Westphal SG, Mannon RB. Biomarkers of rejection in kidney transplantation. Am J Kidney Dis. 2025;85(3):364–74. https://doi.org/10.1053/j.ajkd.2024.07.018.
15. Josephson MA. Monitoring and managing graft health in the kidney transplant recipient. Clin J Am Soc Nephrol. 2011;6(7):1774–80. https://doi.org/10.2215/CJN.01230211.
16. Aubert O, Ursule-Dufait C, Brousse R, Gueguen J, Racapé M, Raynaud M, Van Loon E, Pagliazzi A, Huang E, Jordan SC, Chavin KD, Gupta G, Kumar D, Alhamad T, Anand S, Sanchez-Garcia J, Abdalla BA, Hogan J, Garro R, Dadhania DM, Jain P, Mandelbrot DA, Naesens M, Dandamudi R, Dharnidharka VR, Anglicheau D, Lefaucheur C, Loupy A. Cell-free DNA for the detection of kidney allograft rejection. Nat Med. 2024;30(8):2320–7. https://doi.org/10.1038/s41591-024-03087-3.
17. Bu L, Gupta G, Pai A, Anand S, Stites E, Moinuddin I, Bowers V, Jain P, Axelrod DA, Weir MR, Wolf-Doty TK, Zeng J, Tian W, Qu K, Woodward R, Dholakia S, De Golovine A, Bromberg JS, Murad H, Alhamad T. Clinical outcomes from the assessing donor-derived cell-free DNA monitoring insights of kidney allografts with longitudinal surveillance (ADMIRAL) study. Kidney Int. 2022;101(4):793–803. https://doi.org/10.1016/j.kint.2021.11.034.
18. Ali H, Mohammed M, Fülöp T, Malik S. Outcomes of thymoglobulin versus basiliximab induction therapies in living donor kidney transplant recipients with mild to moderate immunological risk – a retrospective analysis of UNOS database. Ann Med. 2023;55(1):2215536. https://doi.org/10.1080/07853890.2023.2215536.

19. Jackson AM, Kuperman MB, Montgomery RA. Multiple hyperacute rejections in the absence of detectable complement activation in a patient with endothelial cell reactive antibody. Am J Transplant. 2012;12(6):1643–9. https://doi.org/10.1111/j.1600-6143.2011.03955.x.
20. Sun Q, Cheng Z, Cheng D, Chen J, Ji S, Wen J, Zheng C, Liu Z. De novo development of circulating anti-endothelial cell antibodies rather than pre-existing antibodies is associated with post-transplant allograft rejection. Kidney Int. 2011;79(6):655–62. https://doi.org/10.1038/ki.2010.437.
21. Sánchez-Zapardiel E, Mancebo E, Díaz-Ordoñez M, de Jorge-Huerta L, Ruiz-Martínez L, Serrano A, Castro-Panete MJ, Utrero-Rico A, de Andrés A, Morales JM, Domínguez-Rodríguez S, Paz-Artal E. Isolated De novo Antiendothelial cell antibodies and kidney transplant rejection. Am J Kidney Dis. 2016;68(6):933–43. https://doi.org/10.1053/j.ajkd.2016.07.019.

4 Non-HLA Antibody-Mediated Rejection

Sravanthi Paluri

Case 4.1

Case Study Summary

47-year-old Hispanic female with history of end-stage renal disease (ESRD) due to diabetes mellitus received living related kidney transplant (LRKT) from sister, two haplotypes match, cPRA 0%, she received induction with basiliximab (Simulect); her maintenance included tacrolimus, mycophenolate mofetil, and prednisone. Mycophenolate mofetil dose was reduced after transplant due to being well matched and overall Low immunological risk.

S. Paluri (✉)
Division of Nephrology, Bone and Mineral Metabolism, University of Kentucky, Lexington, KY, USA
e-mail: spa318@uky.edu

H. Fattah, V. Cornea (eds.), *Transplantation in Practice*,
https://doi.org/10.1007/978-3-032-15908-3_4

Post-transplant Clinical Course

- As she was on reduced dose of Immunosuppression she had donor-derived cell-free DNA monitoring (dd-cfDNA) at month 10 which was elevated at 2.2%.
- Donor-specific antibodies checked were negative. AT1-R antibodies were negative too.
- MICA antibody testing in this case was positive. However, MICA genotyping of the donor and recipient was not performed, as both siblings were identical for the classical HLA loci (HLA-A, -B, -C, -DR, -DQ, and -DP). Given that the *MICA gene is located within the major histocompatibility complex (MHC) region*, specifically between the class I (HLA-A, -B, -C) and class II (HLA-DR, -DQ, -DP) loci, it is highly likely that the donor and recipient share identical alleles for MICA as well. Thus, the conclusion was the presence of MICA antibodies in this specific context may not necessarily indicate donor-specific reactivity.
- Throughout the course patient's allograft function otherwise remained stable. Renal allograft biopsy was performed.

Diagnosis

- Suspicious for antibody-mediated rejection based on positive g1 + ptc-2, microvascular inflammation (MVI) -3, (Figs. 4.1, 4.2, and 4.3).
- Mild to Moderate Antibody-mediated rejection based on the molecular microscope assessment (MMDx).

Management Approach

Factors which likely contributed to development of rejection:

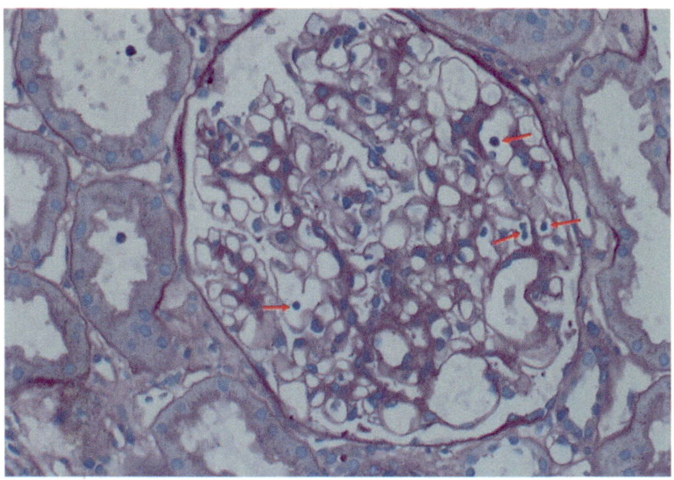

Fig. 4.1 Glomerulitis: capillary loops with intraluminal leukocyte cell infiltrate (red arrows). PAS, 40×

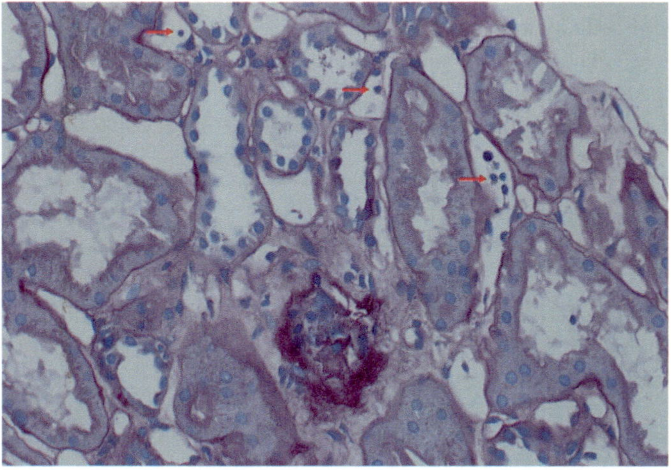

Fig. 4.2 Peritubular capillaritis: Peritubular capillaries with intraluminal leukocyte cell infiltrate (red arrows). PAS, 40×

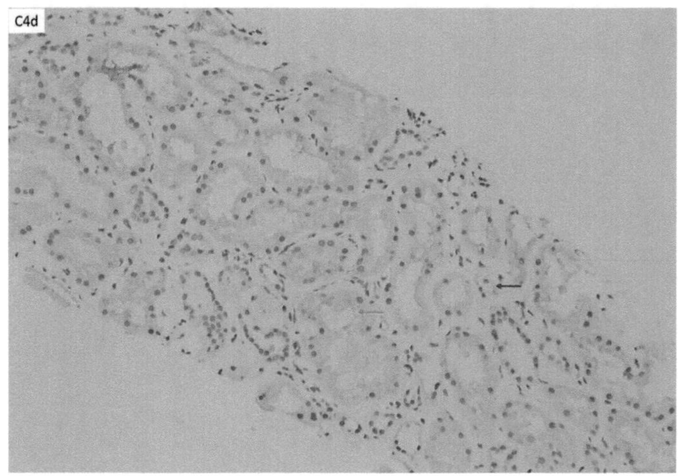

Fig. 4.3 C4d immunostaining: Negative staining in the PTC, (red arrow). Nonspecific cytoplasmic staining in the tubular epithelial cells (blue arrow)

- Basiliximab (Simulect) induction.
- Reduction in immunosuppression (mycophenolate mofetil dose was lowered).
- Possible autoimmune activity due to Non-HLA antibodies.

Treatment

Maximization of maintenance immunosuppression regimen but cell-free DNA remained elevated prompting further addition of fourth immunosuppression agent with bortezomib (Velcade) to target antibody-producing plasma cells.

Follow-Up

- Cell-free DNA post 2 cycles of velcade trended down to 1.1%.
- Stable graft function at 2.5 years.

Educational Insight

- *Antibody-mediated rejection (ABMR)* may occur even in well-matched transplant recipients without an accompanying rise in serum creatinine [1].
- This phenomenon can result from auto- or alloimmune responses directed against non-HLA antigens or previously unrecognized cryptic self-antigens [2].
- In this context, *cell-free DNA (dd-cfDNA) monitoring* has emerged as a valuable adjunct to traditional surveillance methods, offering a sensitive and minimally invasive approach for the early detection of subclinical graft injury when compared with conventional protocol biopsies [3, 4].

Pearl 4.1

This case highlights the role of cell-free DNA in the diagnosis of subclinical allograft injury from antibody-mediated rejection, and possible involvement of autoimmune/alloimmune response toward non HLA cryptic antigens.

Case 4.2

Case Study Summary

- 52-year-old white female with history of end-stage renal disease (ESRD) due to diabetes mellitus; she underwent deceased donor kidney transplant (DDKT) from a donor with profile index (KDPI) of 61%, calculated panel reactive antibody (cPRA) 28%, 0/6 HLA-mismatch; she received induction with anti-thymocyte globulin (ATG) and maintenance regimen included tacrolimus, mycophenolate mofetil, and daily prednisone.

Post-transplant Clinical Course

- She had nadir creatinine baseline of 1.8–2. She was diagnosed with early BK nephropathy. Graft function was stable until 1.5-year post-transplant.
- Renal function worsened 18 months post-transplant after initial stability with BK treatment. Patient received a course of virus specific T cell therapy (VST).
- Donor-specific antibodies were negative; however, cell-free DNA was elevated at 1.4% from previous baseline of 0.6% prompting renal biopsy.

Diagnosis

- Biopsy at 18 months post-transplant—light microscopy—chronic T cell-mediated rejection and moderate microvascular inflammation (MVI) score 4- glomerulitis(g)-1 + peritubular capillaritis(ptc)-3 and transplant glomerulopathy consistent with antibody-mediated rejection (AMR) (Fig. 4.4a and b).
- Molecular biopsy assessment noted for mild to moderate fully developed AMR.
- Non-HLA antibodies AT1-R tested were positive with titers of 11.

Management Approach

Factors which likely contributed to development of AMR:

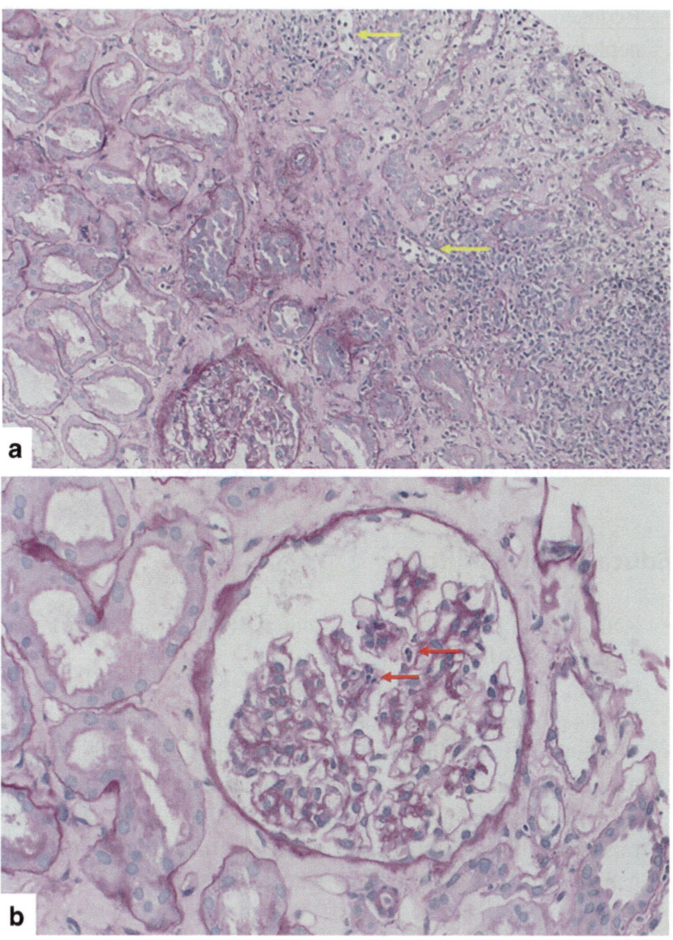

Fig. 4.4 (**a**) Peritubular capillaries with intraluminal leukocytes consistent with peritubular capillaritis (yellow arrows). PAS, 20×. (**b**) Intracapillary glomerular leukocytes consistent with g1 glomerulitis (red arrows). PAS, 40×

- Reduced immunosuppression for earlier diagnosed BK nephropathy.
- Viral specific T cell therapy received for BK nephropathy precipitating rejection.

Treatment:

- Received steroids, Angiotensin receptor blocker (ARB)-Losartan, immunosuppression intensification followed by velcade therapy directed toward antibody-producing plasma cells.

Follow-Up

- Allograft function remained stable with CKD stages 3b-4.

Educational Insights

- Reduction in Immunosuppression for BK nephropathy triggers de novo DSA formation [5].
- Human polyomavirus BKV infection of endothelial cells results in interferon pathway induction [6].
- While there is no direct evidence to suggest BK nephropathy triggers Non-HLA alloimmunity or autoimmunity, there is evidence for Graft injury exposing endothelial antigens [1] and raising the biologic plausibility for BK virus nephropathy triggering Non-HLA antibody-mediated rejection.
- Treatment for non-HLA ABMR is modeled after HLA ABMR management but tailored depending on the specific antibody mechanism [7].

Pearl 4.2

BK nephropathy-related graft injury exposes endothelial polymorphic antigens triggering non HLA alloimmunity and antibody-mediated rejection in well-matched HLA patients.

Case 4.3

Case Study Summary

- 65-year-old White male with history of end-stage renal disease (ESRD) secondary to diabetes mellitus (DM) underwent living unrelated kidney transplant (LUKT), he was not sensitized with cPRA 2%, 5/6 antigen mismatch, received induction with Anti-thymocyte globulin (ATG). Maintenance immunosuppression with tacrolimus, mycophenolate mofetil (MMF) and prednisone.

Post-transplant Clinical Course

- He had protocol donor derived cell-free DNA (dd -cfDNA) trend was noted to be elevated <0.12 to 0.6 at 4 months post-transplant in the setting of reduced Immunosuppression for leucopenia. He was treated for subclinical TCMR with pulse steroids with cell-free DNA down to 0.12.
- He developed BK viremia/BK nephropathy 10 months post-transplant requiring reduction in Immunosuppression.
- 1-year post transplant had rising creatinine and cell-free DNA elevation to 1.5% prompting renal biopsy,
- Donor-specific antibodies checked concomitantly was negative.

Diagnosis

- Light microscopy (Fig. 4.5a and b)—Borderline changes suspicious for Acute T cell-mediated rejection. C4d immunohistochemical stain was negative.
- Molecular biopsy assessment (MMDx) revealed Severe Antibody-mediated rejection and mild T cell-mediated rejection.
- Non-HLA serology positive for AT1R antibodies.

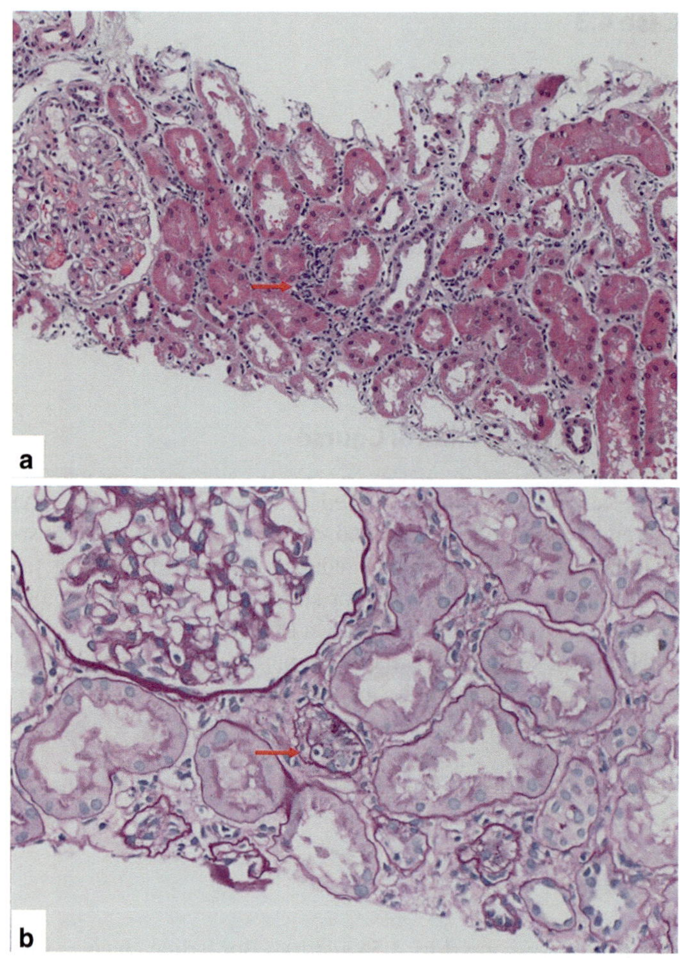

Fig. 4.5 (**a**) Interstitial inflammation (red arrow). H&E, 20×. (**b**). Intraepithelial lymphocytes consistent with tubulitis (red arrow). PAS, 40×

Management Approach

Factors triggering development of antibody-mediated rejection

- Reduction in Immunosuppression for BK viremia, and possibly BK nephritis.

  Treatment approach

- Intensifying immunosuppression, Angiotensin receptor blockers, plasmapheresis, IVIG.

Follow-Up

- Serum creatinine improved with treatment.
- Post-treatment AT1R titers decreased at follow-up.
- Stable graft function 4.5 years from transplant.

Educational Insights

- Reduction in immunosuppression for BK viremia triggers alloimmunity [5].
- The discrepancy between negative histology and positive molecular or cell-free DNA findings in renal allografts can reflect the patchy and evolving nature of antibody-mediated endothelial injury, where molecular injury often precedes or outlasts morphologic changes, or involves subthreshold or non-HLA–driven endothelial activation not captured by Banff criteria. This highlights the clinical relevance of molecular microscope analysis and cell-free DNA testing not only for early detection of subclinical antibody-mediated rejection but also for prognostication, as these tools identify ongoing alloimmune injury and predict future graft dysfunction even in the absence of histologic evidence [8, 9].

- DSA-negative molecularly diagnosed antibody-mediated rejection (mABMR) is more often C4d-negative; diagnosed earlier by 1.5 years (average 2.4 vs. 3.9 years); and had lower ABMR activity and earlier stage in molecular and histology features in comparison to DSA positive ABMR [8].
- ABMR with or without donor-specific antibody in kidney transplants have similar mechanisms and outcomes and hence treatment options remain the same [10].

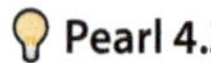

Pearl 4.3

DSA negative molecularly defined antibody-mediated rejection(mABMR) has lower activity in histological features and is more often c4d negative but have identical ABMR-associated transcripts similar to DSA positive mABMR.

Case 4.4

Case Study Summary

- 55-year-old female with end-stage renal disease (ESRD) secondary to polycystic kidney disease. She underwent 0/6 HLA-mismatched deceased donor kidney transplant (DDKT). She was sensitized with calculated PRA of 70%. She received immunosuppression induction with anti-thymocyte globulin (ATG), and maintenance regimen included tacrolimus, mycophenolate mofetil, and daily prednisone.

Post-transplant Clinical Course

- Four months post-transplant, her renal allograft function was stable with serum creatinine of 1.0; however, a donor-derived cell-free DNA (dd-cfDNA) done for surveillance of allograft injury came back elevated at 2%. No HLA donor-specific antibodies were detected.
- Renal allograft biopsy was performed.

Diagnosis

- Biopsy revealed acute T-cell-mediated rejection (TCMR) Banff grade IIA (Fig. 4.6) and active antibody-mediated rejection (ABMR) rejection (Fig. 4.7).
- Molecular biopsy assessment (MMDx) confirmed moderate T-cell-mediated rejection (TCMR) and fully developed antibody-mediated rejection (ABMR).
- Workup for non-HLA antibodies revealed the presence of angiotensin type 1 receptor (AT1R) antibodies.

Management Strategy

- Rabbit anti-thymocyte globulin (rATG) and steroids.
- Maximization of maintenance immunosuppression.
- Received one cycle of Bortezomib.
- Angiotensin receptor blocker was started for positive angiotensin type 1 receptor (AT1R) antibodies.

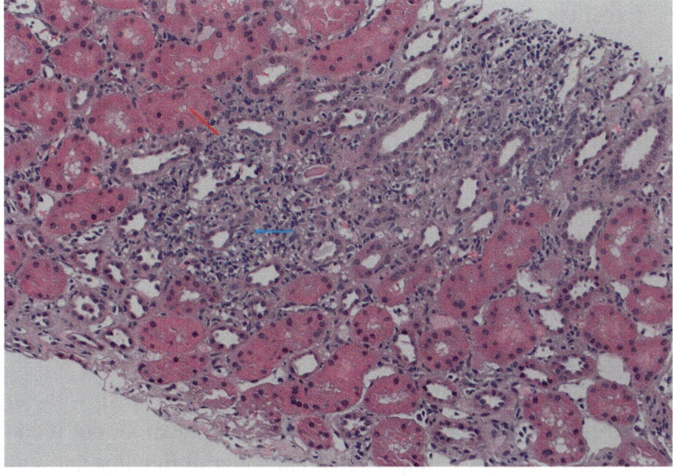

Fig. 4.6 Interstitial inflammation (red arrow), tubulitis (blue arrow). H&E, 20×

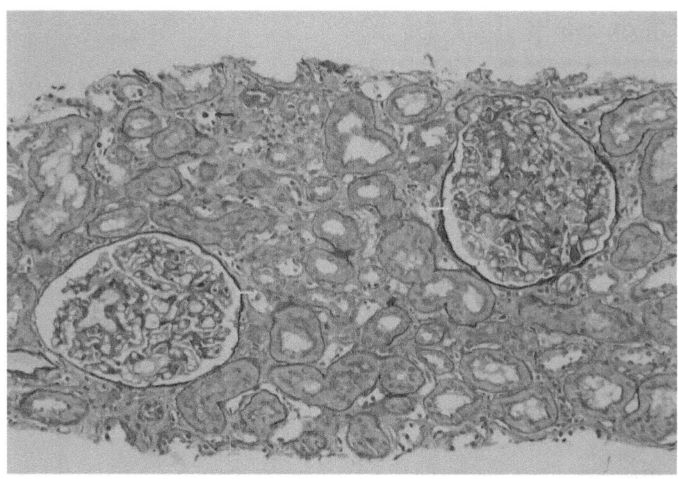

Fig. 4.7 Peritubular capillaritis (red arrows) and glomerulitis (yellow arrows). PAS, 20×

Follow-Up and Prognosis

- Excellent response to treatment. Renal allograft function remains stable at 5 years post-transplant.

Educational Insights

- Most cases of antibody-mediated rejection (ABMR) are thought to be a result of circulating, anti-HLA donor-specific antibodies (DSAs). However, there is evidence to suggest that non-HLA antibodies like the antiangiotensin II type 1 receptor antibodies (AT1R-Ab) also contribute to allograft rejection [11].
- The presence of AT1R-Ab is not only associated with an increased risk of different phenotypes of rejection, but it can also have a negative impact on renal allograft function and survival [12].

- Studies have shown the utility of plasmapheresis, IVIG, immunosuppressive drugs, bortezomib, and rituximab in the treatment of non-HLA antibody-mediated rejection; however, larger clinical trials are needed to confirm the effectiveness of different therapeutic modalities [10].
- Angiotensin receptor blockers, like losartan and candesartan are commonly used in AT1R-Ab-mediated AMR to restrict the interaction between AT1R and antibodies [10, 13].

Pearl 4.4

The presence of AT1R antibodies in kidney transplant recipients is associated with increased risk of rejection and graft loss.

Note: This chapter was authored by Dr. Sravanthi Paluri. It has been reviewed and edited by Dr. Hasan Fattah, the principal author, to maintain consistency with the rest of the book.

References

1. Zhang Q, Reed EF. The importance of non-HLA antibodies in transplantation. Nat Rev Nephrol. 2016;12(8):484–95. https://doi.org/10.1038/nrneph.2016.88.
2. Senev A, Coemans M, Lerut E, Van Sandt V, Daniëls L, Kuypers D, Sprangers B, Emonds MP, Naesens M. Histological picture of antibody-mediated rejection without donor-specific anti-HLA antibodies: clinical presentation and implications for outcome. Am J Transplant. 2019;19(3):763–80. https://doi.org/10.1111/ajt.15074.
3. Bloom RD, Bromberg JS, Poggio ED, Bunnapradist S, Langone AJ, Sood P, Matas AJ, Mehta S, Mannon RB, Sharfuddin A, Fischbach B, Narayanan M, Jordan SC, Cohen D, Weir MR, Hiller D, Prasad P, Woodward RN, Grskovic M, Sninsky JJ, Yee JP, Brennan DC. Circulating donor-derived cell-free DNA in blood for diagnosing active rejection in kidney transplant recipients (DART) study investigators. Cell-free DNA and active rejection in kidney allografts. J Am Soc Nephrol. 2017;28(7):2221–32. https://doi.org/10.1681/ASN.2016091034.
4. Aubert O, Ursule-Dufait C, Brousse R, Gueguen J, Racapé M, Raynaud M, Van Loon E, Pagliazzi A, Huang E, Jordan SC, Chavin KD, Gupta G, Kumar D, Alhamad T, Anand S, Sanchez-Garcia J, Abdalla BA, Hogan J, Garro R, Dadhania DM, Jain P, Mandelbrot DA, Naesens M, Dandamudi

R, Dharnidharka VR, Anglicheau D, Lefaucheur C, Loupy A. Cell-free DNA for the detection of kidney allograft rejection. Nat Med. 2024;30(8):2320–7. https://doi.org/10.1038/s41591-024-03087-3.

5. Moest WT, de Vries APJ, Roelen DL, Kers J, Moes DAR, van der Helm D, Mallat MJK, Meziyerh S, van Rijn AL, Feltkamp MCW, Rotmans JI. BK polyomavirus DNAemia with a high DNA load is associated with De novo donor-specific HLA antibodies in kidney transplant recipients. J Med Virol. 2024;96(11):e70084. https://doi.org/10.1002/jmv.70084.
6. An P, Sáenz Robles MT, Duray AM, Cantalupo PG, Pipas JM. Human polyomavirus BKV infection of endothelial cells results in interferon pathway induction and persistence. PLoS Pathog. 2019;15(1):e1007505. https://doi.org/10.1371/journal.ppat.1007505.
7. Dragun D, Müller DN, Bräsen JH, Fritsche L, Nieminen-Kelhä M, Dechend R, Kintscher U, Rudolph B, Hoebeke J, Eckert D, Mazak I, Plehm R, Schönemann C, Unger T, Budde K, Neumayer HH, Luft FC, Wallukat G. Angiotensin II type 1-receptor activating antibodies in renal-allograft rejection. N Engl J Med. 2005;352(6):558–69. https://doi.org/10.1056/NEJMoa035717.
8. Sellarés J, Reeve J, Loupy A, Mengel M, Sis B, Skene A, de Freitas DG, Kreepala C, Hidalgo LG, Famulski KS, Halloran PF. Molecular diagnosis of antibody-mediated rejection in human kidney transplants. Am J Transplant. 2013;13(4):971–83. https://doi.org/10.1111/ajt.12150.
9. Halloran PF, Reeve J, Madill-Thomsen KS, Demko Z, Prewett A, Billings P. The trifecta study: comparing plasma levels of donor-derived cell-free DNA with the molecular phenotype of kidney transplant biopsies. J Am Soc Nephrol. 2022;33(2):387–400. https://doi.org/10.1681/ASN.2021091191.
10. Kardol-Hoefnagel T, Otten HG. A comprehensive overview of the clinical relevance and treatment options for antibody-mediated rejection associated with non-HLA antibodies. Transplantation. 2021;105(7):1459–70. https://doi.org/10.1097/TP.0000000000003551.
11. Cardinal H, Dieudé M, Hébert MJ. The emerging importance of non-HLA autoantibodies in kidney transplant complications. J Am Soc Nephrol. 2017;28(2):400–6. https://doi.org/10.1681/ASN.2016070756.
12. Sorohan BM, Baston C, Tacu D, Bucşa C, Ţincu C, Vizireanu P, Sinescu I, Constantinescu I. Non-HLA antibodies in kidney transplantation: immunity and genetic insights. Biomedicine. 2022;10(7):1506. https://doi.org/10.3390/biomedicines10071506.
13. Carroll RP, Riceman M, Hope CM, Zeng A, Deayton S, Bennett GD, Coates PT. Angiotensin II type-1 receptor antibody (AT1Rab) associated humoral rejection and the effect of peri operative plasma exchange and candesartan. Hum Immunol. 2016;77(12):1154–8. https://doi.org/10.1016/j.humimm.2016.08.009.

De Novo Post-transplant Glomerulonephritis

5

Hasan Fattah

Case 5.1

Case Study Summary

Patient: A 25-year-old male with a history of congenital heart disease, who received orthotopic heart transplant (OHT), this was later complicated by calcineurin inhibitor (CNI)-associated end-stage renal disease (ESRD).

Transplant course: He received a deceased donor kidney transplant (DDKT), induction treatment with ATG and steroids.

Post-transplant Clinical Course

- Stable heart and renal function on CNI-based regimen, mycophenolate mofetil, and prednisone.
- He subsequently developed intermittent hematuria associated with mild proteinuria, mostly noticeable during recurrent episodes of acute respiratory infection from previously diagnosed chronic bronchiectasis.

H. Fattah (✉)
Jacob School of Medicine and Biomedical Science,
University at Buffalo, Buffalo, NY, USA

H. Fattah, V. Cornea (eds.), *Transplantation in Practice*,
https://doi.org/10.1007/978-3-032-15908-3_5

- Approximately 10 years post-transplant, proteinuria became persistent and increased significantly, reaching 8 g/g based on a random urine protein-to-creatinine ratio (UPCR).
- The patient had no detectable donor-specific antibodies (DSA) and maintained stable renal function with a serum creatinine of 0.8 mg/dL and an estimated glomerular filtration rate (eGFR) of 100 mL/min/1.73m^2.

Diagnosis

- Renal biopsy revealed mesangial IgA and C3 deposition on immunofluorescence without C1q, consistent with de novo versus secondary IgA nephropathy (Figs. 5.1, 5.2, 5.3, and 5.4).
- There was no histologic evidence of acute or chronic rejection.

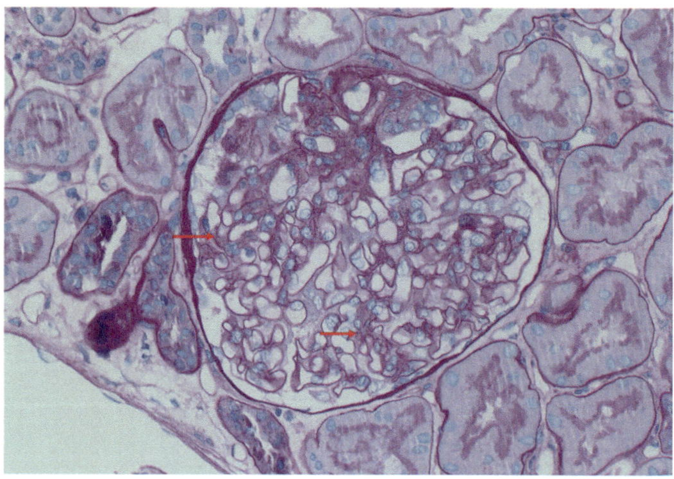

Fig. 5.1 Minimal mesangial matrix expansion (red arrow). PAS, 40×

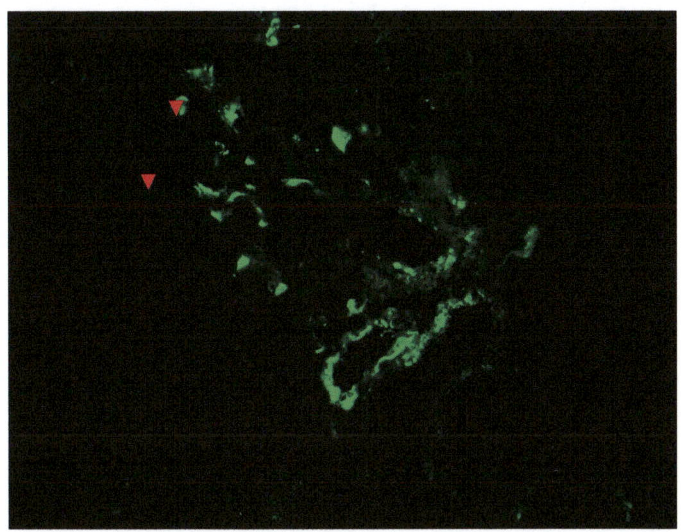

Fig. 5.2 3 + granular mesangial staining (red arrows). IF. C3, 40×

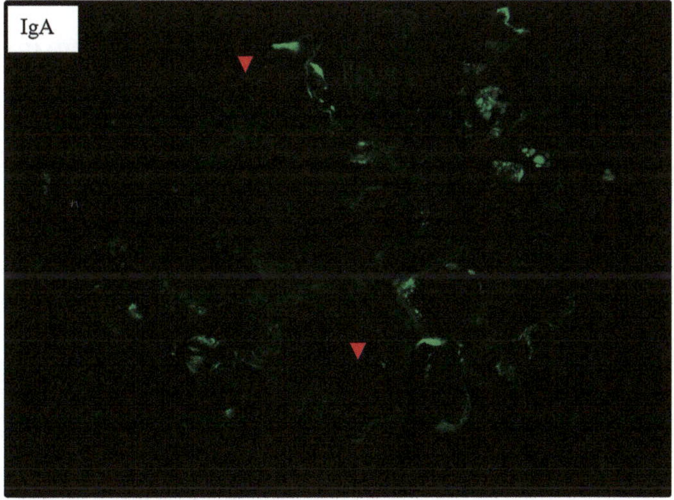

Fig. 5.3 3 + granular mesangial staining (red arrows). IF. IgA, 40×

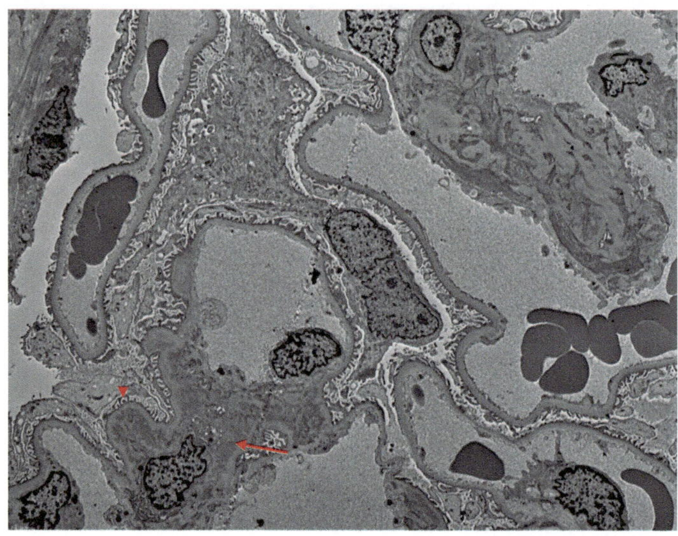

Fig. 5.4 Mesangial electron dense deposits (red arrow). EM, 500×

Management Approach

Potential Triggers and Pathogenesis

- Recurrent respiratory tract infections.
- The case supports a possible mucosa-kidney axis like the pathogenesis in primary IgA nephropathy.
- Immunopathologic findings—mesangial C3 deposition without C1q—suggest activation of the alternative complement pathway.
- There are no definitive histologic features that distinguish primary from secondary IgA nephropathy in transplant recipients.

Medical Treatment

- Angiotensin receptor blockers (ARB) and sodium glucose transport protein 2 inhibitors (SGLT2) were added.
- Antibiotics for the treatment of recurrent bronchitis.

Case Follow-Up

- The patient's kidney allograft function remained stable.
- Serial follow-up random UPCR decreased to 1.5 g/g.

Educational Insights

Mucosa-Kidney Axis in Post-transplant IgA Nephropathy

Like primary IgA nephropathy, the interaction between mucosal immune stimulation (e.g., recurrent respiratory infections) and glomerular IgA deposition may play a role in the development of de novo or secondary IgA nephropathy in kidney transplant recipients.

Complement Pathway Activation

The presence of mesangial C3 deposits without accompanying C1q suggests activation of the alternative complement pathway, which may contribute to disease progression and may have diagnostic or therapeutic implications [1].

Histologic Overlap Between Primary and Secondary IgA Nephropathy

Currently, there are no specific histologic features that reliably distinguish primary from secondary IgA nephropathy. Diagnosis often depends on clinical context, including triggers (e.g., infections), disease timing (e.g., post-transplant), and associated comorbidities.

Importance of Monitoring Proteinuria in Long-Term Graft Surveillance

- A gradual increase in proteinuria—even in the setting of stable graft function—should prompt evaluation for glomerular disease recurrence or de novo glomerular pathology.
- Early intervention can help preserve graft function.

Role of Adjunctive Therapies

Use of renin-angiotensin system (RAS) blockers, endothelin receptor antagonists in addition to SGLT2 inhibitors, may help reduce proteinuria and slow progression [2], although evidence in transplant population is still emerging.

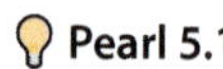

De novo *or secondary IgA nephropathy can develop post-transplant, often triggered by mucosal immune stimulation such as recurrent respiratory infections. Despite stable graft function, rising proteinuria warrants investigation. Mesangial C3 without C1q suggests alternative complement activation, and histology alone may not distinguish primary from secondary forms.*

Case 5.2

Case Study Summary

Patient: A 39-year-old White male with a history of end-stage renal disease (ESRD) secondary to reported chronic glomerulonephritis (GN) of unclear etiology.

Transplant course: He underwent a living-related kidney transplant (LRKT) from his brother approximately 10 years prior to current presentation.

Post-transplant Clinical Course

- The patient presented with progressive deterioration in renal function and nephrotic-range proteinuria, with a random urine protein-to-creatinine ratio (UPCR) of 10 g/g.
- Immunologic Evaluation: Positive antinuclear antibody (ANA) at a titer of 1:80 with a speckled pattern. PLA2R antibody testing was below the diagnostic threshold.
- Comprehensive workup was largely unremarkable, including tests for donor-specific antibodies (DSA), and ddcfDNA.

Diagnosis

De novo idiopathic membranous nephropathy (IMN) presumed primary in nature based on light microscopy, IF, and EM (Figs. 5.5, 5.6, and 5.7).

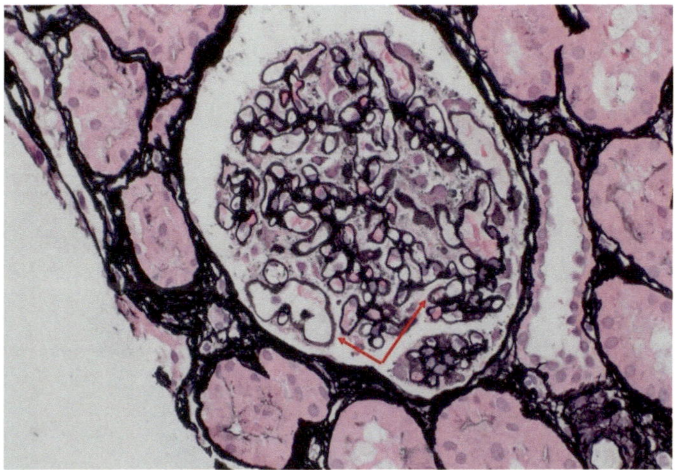

Fig. 5.5 Characteristic spikes of basement membrane (red arrows). Jones silver stain, 40×

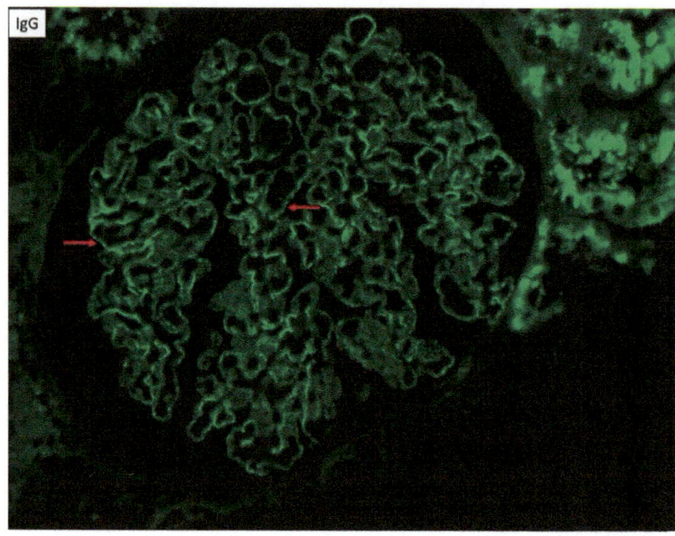

Fig. 5.6 IgG granular staining in the capillary walls (red arrow), IF, 40×

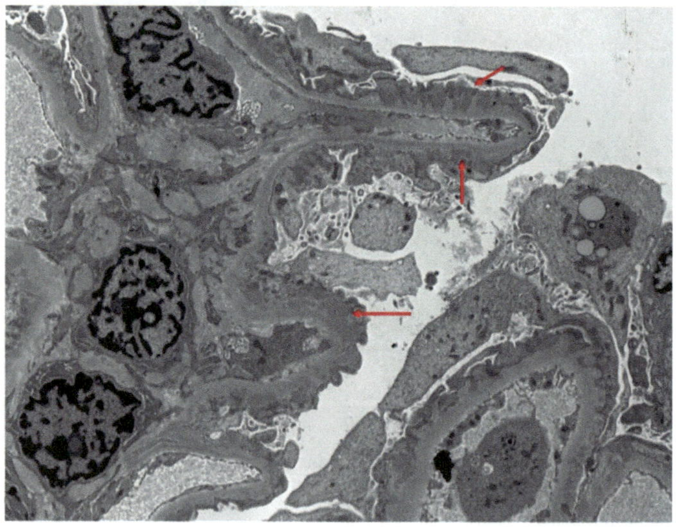

Fig. 5.7 Subepithelial electron dense deposits (red arrow). EM, 1200×

Management Approach

- Follow-up malignancy screening, and infectious etiologies were unrevealing.
- Potential contributing factors:
  - Genetic predisposition and shared HLA antigens due to living-related donation [3].
  - Possible under-immunosuppression over time.
- Initiated on angiotensin receptor blockers (ARBs).
- Received rituximab (anti-CD20 monoclonal antibody) therapy.

Case Follow-Up

The patient achieved complete remission with stable allograft function maintained over a 2-year period since most recent follow-up visit.

Educational Insights

Recurrent vs. de novo *membranous nephropathy*: Membranous nephropathy (MN) post-transplant may represent either recurrence of a native disease or a de novo process. Both forms can manifest at any time following transplantation.

Prevalence and impact: Recurrent clinical and subclinical iMN occurs in approximately 48% of cases and poses a significant risk to graft survival [4].

Therapeutic implications: in addition to conventional use of ARB or ACEi the early and progressive iMN post-transplant responds well to B-cell depletion therapy (e.g., rituximab), with many patients achieving clinical and histological remission [5].

Pearl 5.2

Membranous nephropathy (MN) after kidney transplantation can be either recurrent or de novo *and may present early or many years post-transplant. Early recognition and treatment with anti-*

CD20 therapy can lead to both clinical and histological remission. Risk factors may include genetic predisposition—especially in living-related donors—and under-immunosuppression, highlighting the need for long-term vigilance in transplant recipients.

Case 5.3

Case Study Summary

Patient: A 34-year-old male with end-stage renal disease (ESRD) of unknown etiology.

Transplant course: He received a deceased donor kidney transplant (DDKT) from a donor with a kidney donor profile index (KDPI) of 3%. The graft was well-matched, and the patient was non-sensitized at the time of transplant. Induction treatment with ATG and steroids, maintained on standard triple therapy: tacrolimus, mycophenolate mofetil (MMF), and prednisone.

Post-transplant clinical course: Patient developed new-onset nephrotic-range proteinuria (random urine protein to creatinine ratio UPCR of 5 g/g) without hematuria approximately 1 year after transplant. Serologic, rejection molecular, and infectious workup failed to reveal any abnormalities.

Diagnosis

Kidney biopsy: C1q nephropathy as revealed on biopsy with findings of severe interstitial fibrosis and tubular atrophy (IFTA) in (Fig. 5.8) with prominent mesangial C1q and IgM deposits on IF (Fig. 5.9a and b). Electron microscopy showed patchy podocyte foot process effacement, without any features suggestive of classic immune complex glomerulonephritis (Fig. 5.10).

Final pathology diagnosis: C1q nephropathy (C1qN) in the transplanted kidney.

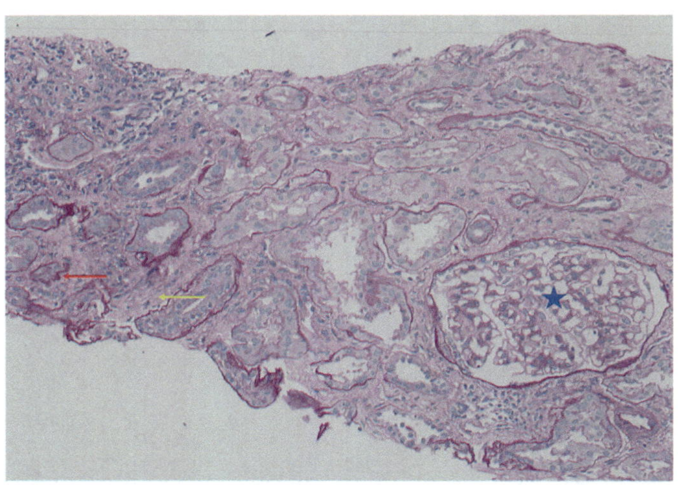

Fig. 5.8 Interstitial fibrosis (yellow arrow), tubular atrophy (red arrow), and normocellular glomeruli (blue star), PAS, 20×

Management Approach

Presumed triggering factors: Unclear; no evidence of recent infection, donor-derived disease, or immunologic sensitization.

Treatment: Initiated on angiotensin receptor blockers (ARBs) and sodium-glucose cotransporter 2 (SGLT2) inhibitors for anti-proteinuric effect.

Follow-Up

- At 3 years follow-up visit, the patient maintains stable graft function and has achieved complete remission of proteinuria while on dual therapy with ARBs and SGLT2 inhibitors and adequate maintenance immunosuppression.

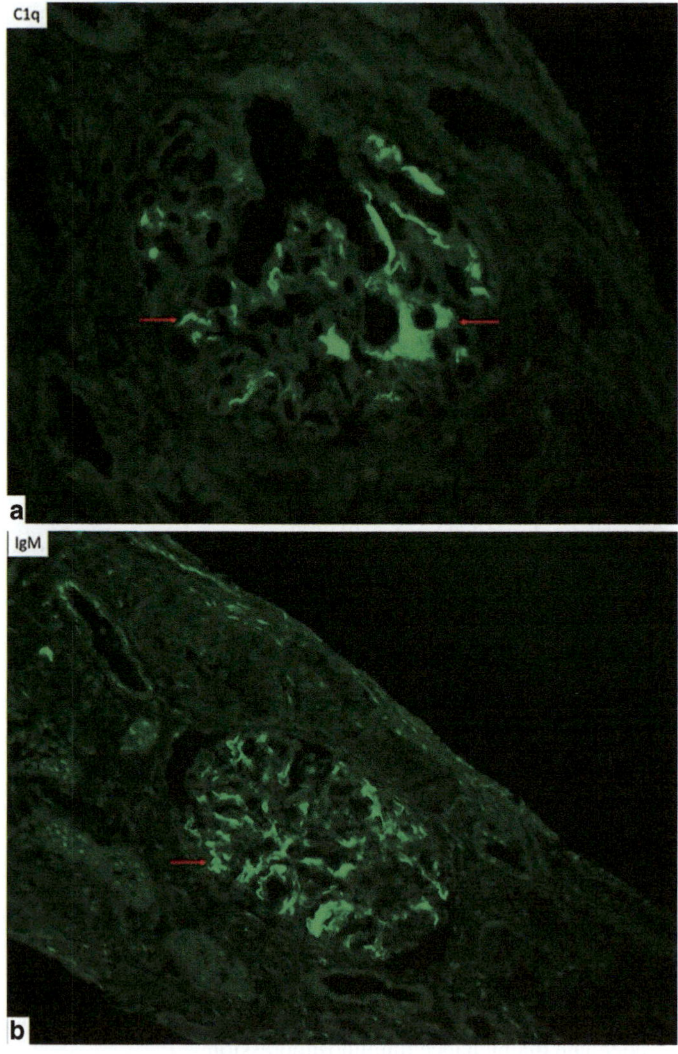

Fig. 5.9 (**a**) 2+ mesangial granular staining for C1q. IF, 40× (**b**) 2+ granular mesangial staining for IgM, IF, 40×

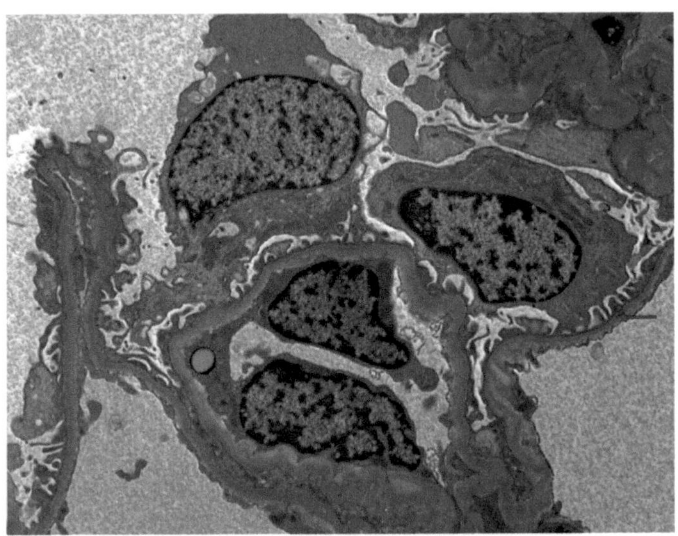

Fig. 5.10 Insignificant foot process effacement (discrete foot process, red arrow). EM, 1200×

Educational Insights

- C1q nephropathy (C1qN) is a rare and mostly benign findings seen on protocol biopsies and only rarely presents with proteinuria or histologic features such as focal segmental glomerulosclerosis like in our case [6].
- It is characterized by dominant or codominant mesangial C1q deposition on immunofluorescence. The exact pathogenesis remains unclear. Specialized C1q receptors located on mesangial cells are thought to play a role by facilitating the binding and trapping of immune complexes within the glomerulus, possibly triggered by circulating antigens (such as viral ones) or in situ antigen formation.
- An alternative hypothesis suggests that C1q may nonspecifically bind to immunoglobulins and become secondarily entrapped in the paramesangial region, particularly in the context of increased mesangial trafficking, as seen in proteinuric states.

- Approximately half of the reported cases are preceded by infections, suggesting that C1q nephropathy may represent an atypical or post-infectious glomerulonephritis in some patients. Certain viral agents, including Epstein-Barr virus (EBV) and BK virus, have been tentatively associated with the disease [7].

Pearl 5.3

C1q nephropathy is a rare cause of post-transplant proteinuria, marked by dominant mesangial C1q deposits. Its pathogenesis may involve immune complexes or nonspecific trapping in proteinuric states. Viral infections like EBV or BK virus are possible triggers, though C1q deposits can sometimes be incidental in allografts without clinical impact.

Case 5.4

Case Study Summary

Patient: A 36-year-old male with end-stage renal disease (ESRD) of unknown etiology.

Transplant course: he underwent a living unrelated kidney transplant (LUKT) with an initially uneventful post-operative course. Maintenance home medications consist of Tacrolimus, Azathioprine, and daily dose of 5 mg prednisone.

Post-transplant Clinical Course

- Five years after transplant, he developed nephrotic-range proteinuria and microscopic hematuria.
- Serologic workup was largely unremarkable.
- ANA was positive at a low titer.
- Donor-specific antibodies (DSAs) were detected against the HLA-DR antigen with a mean fluorescence intensity (MFI) of 3000.

- Kidney Biopsy: Revealed necrotizing glomerulonephritis with dominant mesangial IgA deposition on immunofluorescence, consistent with de novo IgA nephropathy.

Diagnosis

Necrotizing glomerulonephritis with predominant IgA glomerular staining (Figs. 5.11 and 5.12).

Management Approach

Presumed triggering factor: Reduced immunosuppression over time, community acquired viral and bacterial infections may have contributed to disease activation.

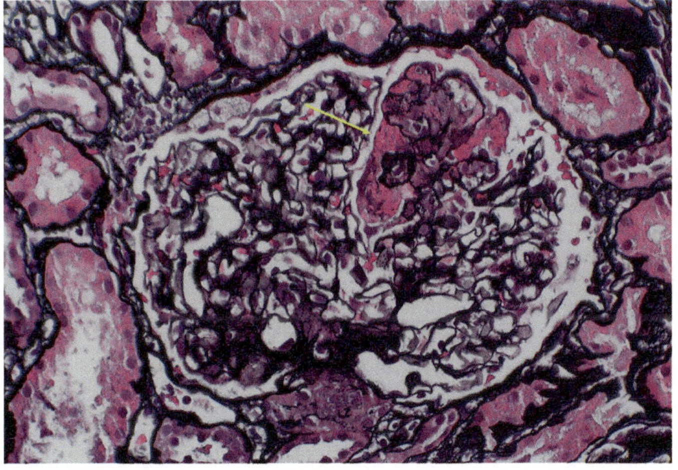

Fig. 5.11 Basement membrane breaks and fibrin deposition (yellow arrow). Jones silver stain, 40×

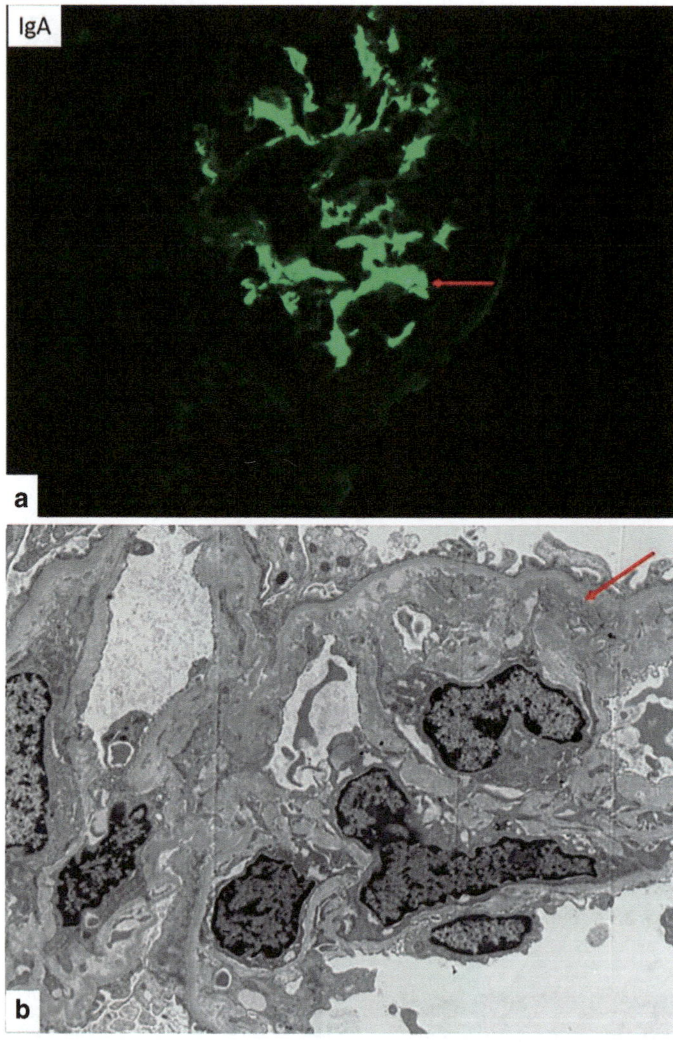

Fig. 5.12 (**a**) IgA mesangial staining picture (red arrow). IF 40×. (**b**) mesangial immune complex deposits (red arrow). EM 1200×

Treatment:

- Initiated on oral corticosteroids.
- Azathioprine was replaced with mycophenolate mofetil (MMF) to enhance immunosuppression.
- Supportive therapy with angiotensin receptor blockers (ARBs) and SGLT2 inhibitors.

Follow-Up

- Partial remission of proteinuria was achieved, and graft function remains stable throughout years of follow-up.

Educational Insights

- necrotizing glomerulonephritis with predominant IgA staining after kidney transplant most commonly represents recurrent or de novo IgA nephropathy or IgA-dominant post-infectious glomerulonephritis (PIGN).
- careful integration of clinical, serologic, and detailed immunofluorescence findings is essential for accurate diagnosis and differentiation from C1q nephropathy and other post-transplant glomerular diseases [8].
- De novo IgA nephropathy may be triggered by infections and could present in its aggressive form with necrotizing lesions and more severe glomerular injury, as seen in this case. Reduced immunosuppression may unmask or exacerbate such immune responses.

Pearl 5.4

Necrotizing glomerulonephritis with dominant IgA staining post-transplant often indicates recurrent or de novo *IgA nephropathy, or IgA-dominant post-infectious glomerulonephritis (PIGN).*

Accurate diagnosis requires careful correlation of clinical presentation, serologic data, and detailed immunofluorescence. De novo *IgA nephropathy may be infection-triggered and present aggressively with necrotizing lesions, especially when immunosuppression is reduced.*

Case 5.5

Case Study Summary

Patient: A 19-year-old male with end-stage renal disease (ESRD) secondary to congenital abnormalities of the kidney and urinary tract (CAKUT).

Transplant course: He received a deceased donor kidney transplant (DDKT), induction and maintenance immunosuppression included (ATG), steroids, tacrolimus trough level goals 8–10, and mycophenolate mofetil (MMF) in combination with daily prednisone dose of 5 mg.

Post-transplant Course

- Three months after transplant, the patient developed new-onset sub-nephrotic range proteinuria and microscopic hematuria.
- Initial Workup: Comprehensive evaluation for viral, autoimmune and alloimmune disorders were unrevealing.
- Kidney Biopsy Findings: Unremarkable for rejection, or de novo immune complex deposition per immunofluorescence; however, there were moderate interstitial fibrosis and approximately 50% podocyte foot process effacement noted on electron microscopy.

Diagnosis

Secondary de novo focal segmental glomerulosclerosis (FSGS) as shown on EM (Figs. 5.13 and 5.14).

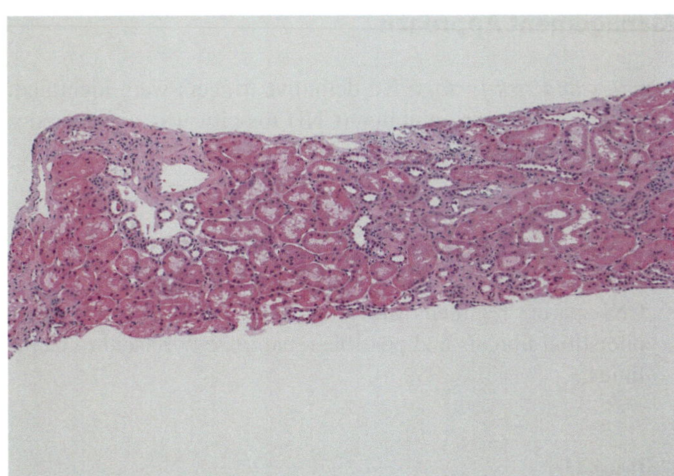

Fig. 5.13 Unremarkable histology, mild to moderate interstitial fibrosis. H&E, 10×

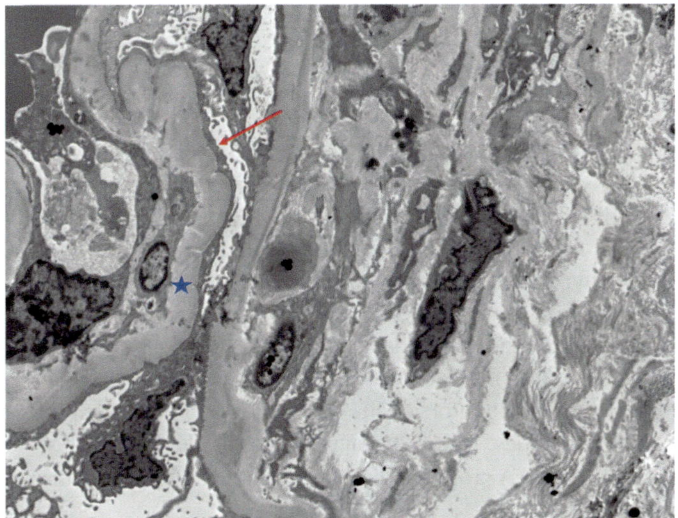

Fig. 5.14 Moderate 50% effacement of foot processes (red arrow), blue star to identify glomerular basement membrane

Management Approach

Triggers and risk factors: No definitive triggers were identified; however, calcineurin inhibitor (CNI) toxicity was considered a possible contributing factor.

Treatment:

- Initiation of angiotensin receptor blocker (ARB) therapy.
- Evaluation to exclude secondary causes of FSGS.
- CNI-sparing regimens were suggested due to early moderate interstitial fibrosis and possible renal toxicity related to tacrolimus.

Follow-Up

- Resolution of proteinuria.
- Maintained stable graft function for years after initial diagnosis.

Educational Insights

- De novo FSGS can manifest after transplant with varying degrees of proteinuria, ranging from mild to nephrotic levels.
- A discrepancy between recipient body mass and the nephron mass of a single transplanted kidney may result in compensatory hyperfiltration, predisposing to podocyte injury and FSGS.
- Secondary causes of FSGS include viral infections, ischemia, drugs, and other conditions leading to nephron loss and increased glomerular stress.
- Calcineurin inhibitors (CNIs) known for their podocyte protective properties, can also contribute to the development of de novo FSGS. A proposed mechanism of this; CNIs may enhance

TGF-β expression in podocytes via increase in reactive oxygen species (ROS), promoting podocyte apoptosis and detachment from the glomerular basement membrane—a known mechanism in the pathogenesis of FSGS [9, 10]. This may present with:

- Progressive proteinuria.
- Hypertension.
- Subtle decline in allograft function.

Pearl 5.5

De novo *FSGS can emerge after transplant as sub-nephrotic or nephrotic-range proteinuria, often without clear triggers. In this case, CNI toxicity was a suspected contributor, highlighting its role in podocyte injury* via *TGF-β-mediated pathways. Recognizing secondary risk factors is crucial for early diagnosis and management to preserve graft function.*

Case 5.6

Case Study Summary

Patient: A 63-year-old female with end-stage renal disease (ESRD) secondary to autosomal dominant polycystic kidney disease (ADPKD).

Transplant course: She underwent a deceased donor kidney transplant (DDKT) with uneventful post-transplant course and stable renal allograft function on traditional treatment included daily prednisone 5 mg, tacrolimus with target trough levels 4–6, and small dose of mycophenolate mofetil (MMF).

Clinical course: During a routine visit with her nephrologist, at around 14 years after transplant, a new-onset proteinuria (UPCR of 1.8 g/g on random spot urine) and microscopic hematuria were noted on her routine lab results. Serum creatinine remained unchanged from known baseline range.

Initial Workup

- Negative for monoclonal gammopathy and alloimmune disorders.
- No recent viral or bacterial infections reported.
- Low serum complements levels (C3 and C4).
- Genetic testing for C3 abnormalities were equivocal.

Diagnosis

De novo C3-dominant glomerulonephritis (C3GN) based on biopsy results, shown as MPGN on H&E (Fig. 5.15), and confirmed on formalin-fixed, paraffin-embedded tissue IF (Fig. 5.16) and EM (Fig. 5.17).

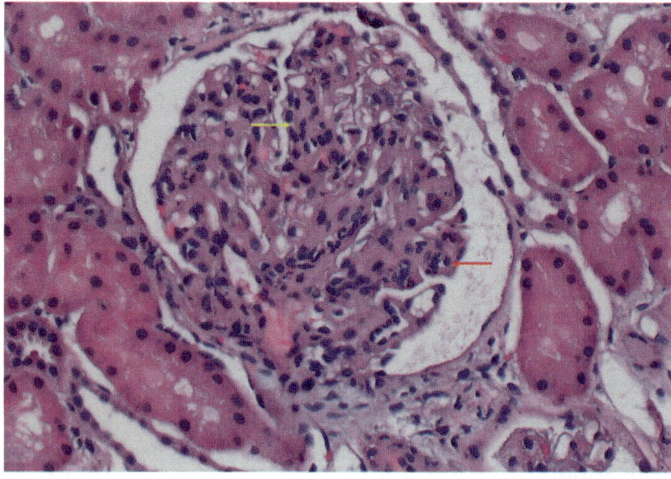

Fig. 5.15 MPGN features, endocapillary (red arrow), and mesangial (yellow arrow) increased cellularity. H&E, 40×

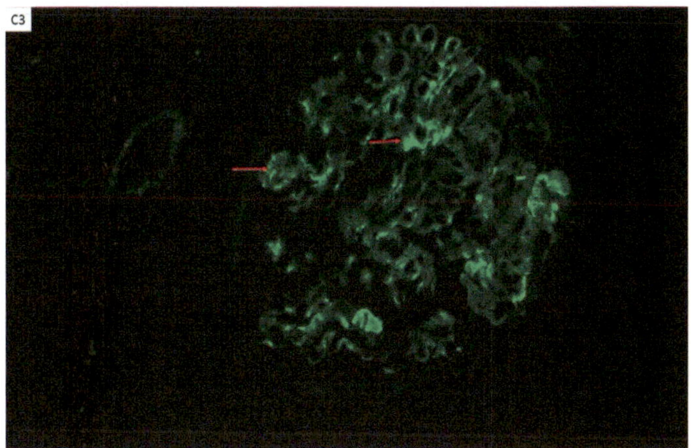

Fig. 5.16 C3 Granular 2+ mesangial staining (red arrow). Immunofluorescence C3, 40×

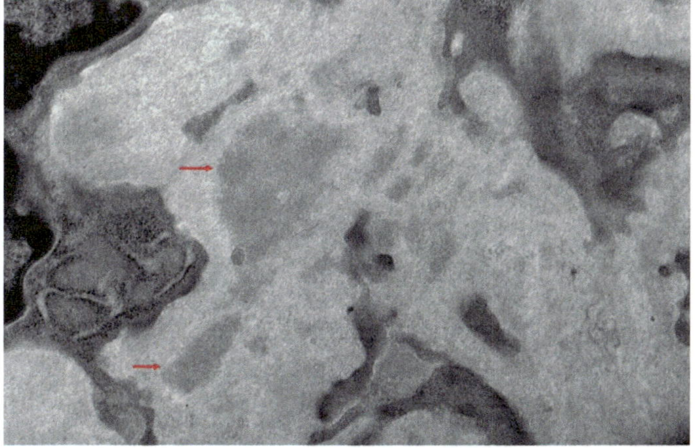

Fig. 5.17 Mesangial electron dense deposits (red arrow), Electron Microscope, 600×

Management Approach

Triggering factors: No clear precipitating factor identified at the time of diagnosis.

Treatment: Initiated treatment with an angiotensin receptor blocker (ARB) to reduce proteinuria, along with evaluation of complement pathway abnormalities.

Follow-Up

- Gradual improvement in proteinuria and hematuria.
- Stable renal allograft function at the most recent follow-up visit.

Educational Insights

- De novo C3 glomerulopathy is a rare disease that presents with post-transplant proteinuria and hematuria, often occurring years after transplantation.
- Prior to confirming a diagnosis of C3 glomerulonephritis (C3GN), it is essential to exclude monoclonal gammopathy, especially those with membranoproliferative (MPGN) patterns on the kidney biopsy. These may yield false-negative results on standard immunofluorescence. Performing immunofluorescence on formalin-fixed, paraffin-embedded tissue after protease digestion can unmask hidden monoclonal immunoglobulin deposits [11].
- A thorough evaluation should also include testing for recent or remote infections, autoantibodies to complement factors (such as C3, C5 nephritic factors), and, if unrevealing, genetic analysis of the alternative complement pathway.

Pearl 5.6

In late post-transplant patients with proteinuria and low complement levels, consider de novo *C3 glomerulonephritis. Always rule out masked monoclonal gammopathy using protease-digested immunofluorescence and assess for infections, complement autoantibodies, and if needed genetic abnormalities to ensure accurate diagnosis.*

Case 5.7

Case Study Summary

Patient: A 54-year-old male with end-stage renal disease (ESRD) of unknown etiology.

Transplant course: He received a pediatric En Bloc kidney transplant. He maintained excellent graft function for 18 years. He later developed acute kidney injury (AKI) and nephrotic-range proteinuria following COVID-19 infection. Evaluation showed no evidence of donor-specific antibodies (DSA) or elevated donor-derived cell-free DNA (dd-cfDNA), other viral serologies and full workup for AKI were all unremarkable.

Diagnosis

Secondary focal segmental glomerulosclerosis (FSGS) following COVID 19 infection, diagnosis is made based on EM (Fig. 5.18) and clinical presentation, features of transplant glomerulopathy (TG) on light microscopy (Fig. 5.19).

Management Approach

Potential Triggers

- Possibly COVID-19 infection.
- Chronic calcineurin inhibitor (CNI) toxicity.

Treatment: Conservative treatment with angiotensin receptor blocker (ARB) and SGLT2 inhibitors.

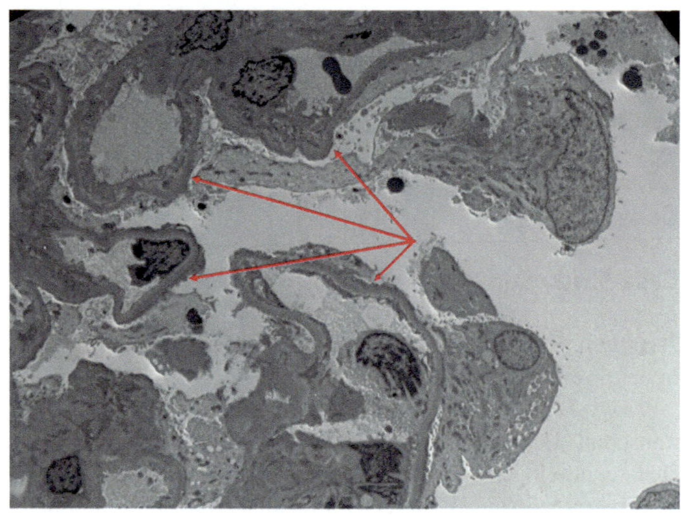

Fig. 5.18 Diffuse effacement of the foot processes (red arrows), EM 500×

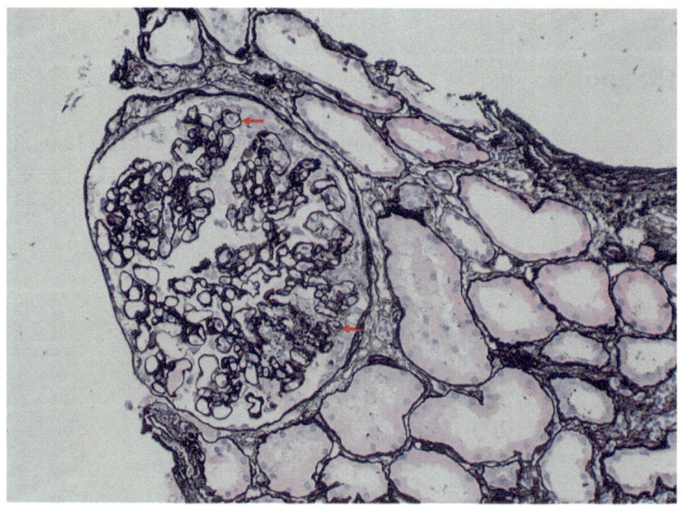

Fig. 5.19 GBM double contours (red arrows), Silver Jones stain, 20×

Follow-Up

Four years post-diagnosis:

- Graft function remains stable at CKD stage 3b.
- Partial remission of proteinuria (urine protein-to-creatinine ratio reduced from 8 to 1 g/g).

Educational Insights

- COVID-19 has been increasingly associated with the onset or relapse of FSGS in the kidneys, including in kidney transplant recipients, most notably the collapsing variant.
- The pathogenesis is thought to involve both direct and indirect mechanisms, via direct podocyte injury and immune dysregulation, respectively [12–14].
- Transplant glomerulopathy (TG) is a common long-term complication of kidney transplantation. Its pathogenesis is multifactorial, involving:
  - Chronic antibody-mediated rejection (ABMR).
  - Cell-mediated immune injury.
  - Podocyte stress from adapting to a "two-kidney-to-one-kidney transition" (as in pediatric en bloc transplants). These mechanisms contribute to a shared pathway of repetitive endothelial injury, leading to glomerular basement membrane duplication and chronic graft dysfunction.

Pearl 5.7

COVID-19 may trigger secondary FSGS in transplant recipients through podocyte injury and immune dysregulation. Transplant glomerulopathy often reflects cumulative endothelial injury from chronic rejection, CNI toxicity, and podocyte stress, especially in long-surviving renal transplant grafts.

Case 5.8

Case Study Summary

Patient: A 62-year-old female with end-stage renal disease (ESRD) secondary to type 1 diabetes mellitus.

Transplant course: She received a simultaneous kidney-pancreas transplant approximately 20 years prior to her presentation, her maintenance treatment included daily dose of prednisone of 5 mg, tacrolimus with target trough levels 4–6, and mycophenolate mofetil.

Clinical course: On presentation she developed classic nephrotic syndrome with preserved renal and pancreatic allograft function.

Diagnosis

Based on biopsy report; idiopathic de novo focal segmental glomerulosclerosis (FSGS) (Figs. 5.20 and 5.21).

Management Approach

Risk factors: No clear precipitating factor identified.

Treatment: Initiated therapy with angiotensin receptors blockers (ARB), oral steroids with minimal improvement. Patient refused plasma exchange. ACTH (repository corticotropin injection) was tried later with satisfactory response.

Follow-Up

- Achieved complete remission of nephrotic syndrome with ACTH and corticosteroids.
- Allograft function remained stable, unfortunately patient developed DM and returned to the use of insulin.

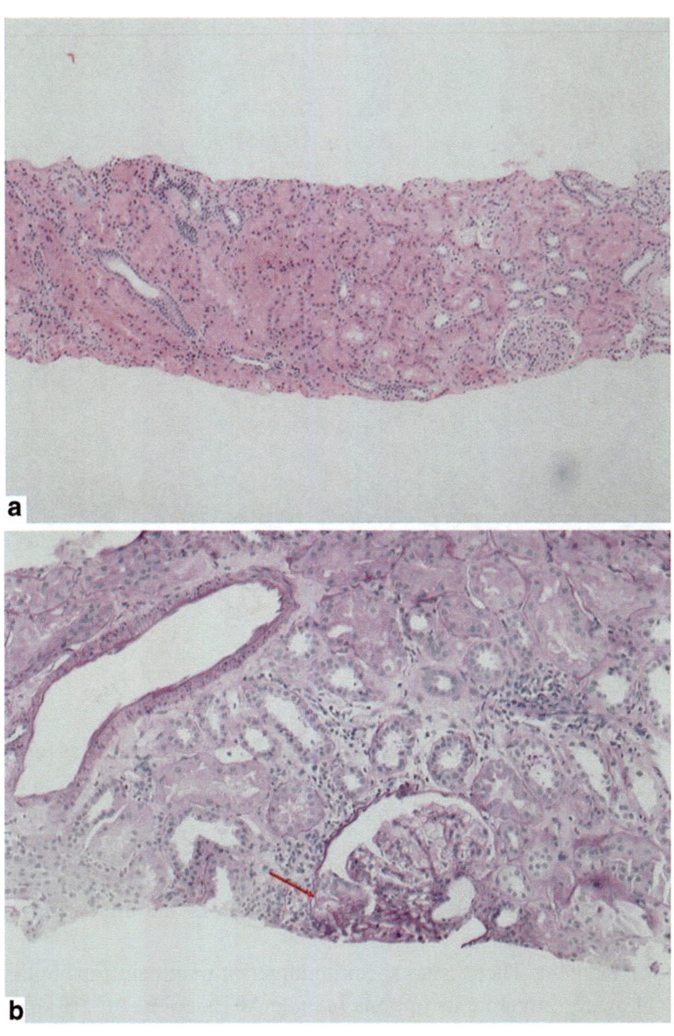

Fig. 5.20 (**a**) No active alloimmune injury. H&E, 10×. (**b**) Segmental glomerular capillary sclerosis (red arrow). PAS, 20×

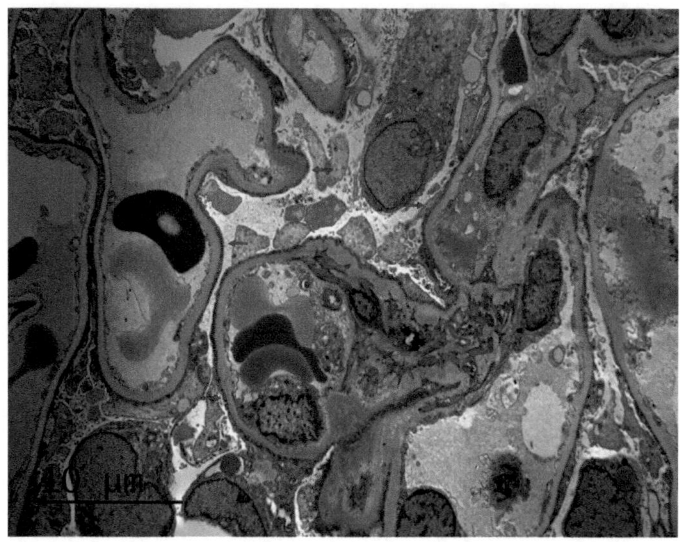

Fig. 5.21 Extensive foot processes effacement (red arrows) on electron microscope

Educational Insights

- De novo FSGS post-kidney transplant can be classified as idiopathic or secondary (e.g., viral infections, medications, anabolic steroids). Idiopathic forms can occur at any time post-transplant, often without a clear trigger.
- Proposed mechanisms for idiopathic de novo FSGS include podocyte injury from calcineurin inhibitors and alloimmune-mediated damage.
- Treatment: There is no specific universal treatment for FSGS; however, treatments options include ACEi, ARB, ACTH [15], steroids, and, in select cases, plasmapheresis (PLEX) with or without rituximab [16].
- Partial or complete remission occurs in 57% of patients and is associated with better graft survival. This is supported by high-quality multicenter cohort data [17].

Pearl 5.8

Idiopathic post-transplant de novo *FSGS can occur years after kidney transplantation without a clear trigger; it can manifest with classic nephrotic syndrome. Though the exact mechanism is unclear, podocyte injury from calcineurin inhibitors and alloimmune responses are proposed contributors. Treatment is not specific; partial or complete remission is associated with better outcomes.*

Case 5.9

Case Study Summary

Patient: A 66-year-old male with ESRD secondary to diabetes mellitus type II.

Transplant course: He received a living-related kidney transplant (LRKT) and maintained stable graft function for several years on traditional treatment included CNI, MMF, and daily prednisone.

Clinical course: In late 2021, he was diagnosed with acute COVID-19 infection, which was complicated by acute kidney injury. Approximately 3 months later, he developed new-onset nephrotic-range proteinuria and microscopic hematuria. His glycemic control remained optimal (A1C 6%), and serologic workup and imaging were unremarkable.

Diagnosis

Based on kidney biopsy: Secondary FSGS, not otherwise specified (NOS) (Fig. 5.22), with underlying diabetic changes.

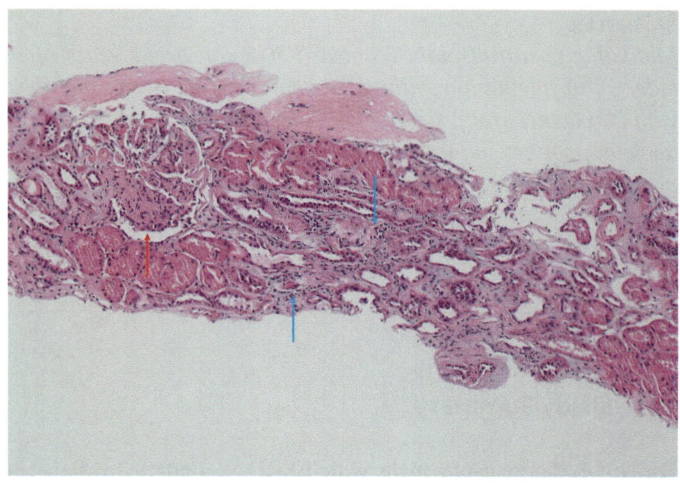

Fig. 5.22 Segmental glomerular scar, red arrow (FSGS) and interstitial fibrosis (blue arrows). H&E, 10×

Management Approach

Potential Triggering Factors

- Recent COVID-19 infection.
- Background of diabetes mellitus.

Treatment: Conservative treatment with angiotensin receptors blockers (ARB) and optimizing medical treatment for HTN and DM.

Follow-Up

The patient experienced a progressive decline in graft function and ultimately initiated dialysis.

Educational Insights

- FSGS has been linked to several viral infections, with HIV-associated collapsing FSGS being the most well-characterized.
- Other viruses implicated in FSGS pathogenesis include parvovirus B19, CMV, EBV, BK, SV40, and hepatitis C. More recently, COVID-19 has been associated with both collapsing and non-collapsing variants of FSGS, particularly in individuals with high-risk APOL1 genotypes.
- Viral infections may induce direct podocyte injury or trigger immune-mediated responses that result in segmental glomerular sclerosis and proteinuria.

Pearl 5.9

Viral infections, including COVID-19, can trigger secondary forms of FSGS in kidney transplant recipients. COVID-19–associated FSGS has been increasingly recognized, particularly in patients with high-risk backgrounds or underlying comorbidities such as diabetes, or high risk APOL1 genotypes. Prompt recognition is important, though outcomes may be poor due to chronic changes and limited treatment options.

Case 5.10

Case Study Summary

Patient: A 24-year-old female with ESRD secondary to congenital abnormalities of kidney and urinary tract (CAKUT).

Transplant course: She received a deceased donor kidney transplant (DDKT) 5 years prior to this presentation.

Clinical presentation: She developed sudden-onset nephrotic-range proteinuria (20 g/g based on multiple random urine protein creatinine ratios), microscopic hematuria (>50 RBCs/HPF), and acute kidney injury (creatinine increased from 0.7 to 4.0 mg/dL).

Laboratory Workup

- Complement levels (C3, C4): Within normal limits.
- Immunologic serologies: dsDNA was detected at a titer of 1:80; ANA, RF, both ANCAs (MPO/PR3), anti-Smith antibodies, and anti-RNP were all undetectable.
- Infectious markers: Negative for HIV, HCV, CMV, BK, B19 and HBV per PCRs methods.
- Immunologic profile: History of poor adherence to immunosuppressive therapy (on azathioprine and tacrolimus), with emergence of multiple donor-specific antibodies (DSA) totaling 80,000 MFI against multiple antigens from across the donor HLA spectrum; dd-cfDNA was not elevated, at 0.1%.

Diagnosis

- De novo diffuse lupus nephritis (class IV-G, A/C) (Figs. 5.23, 5.24, and 5.25) with secondary membranous nephropathy (class V) (Fig. 5.26).

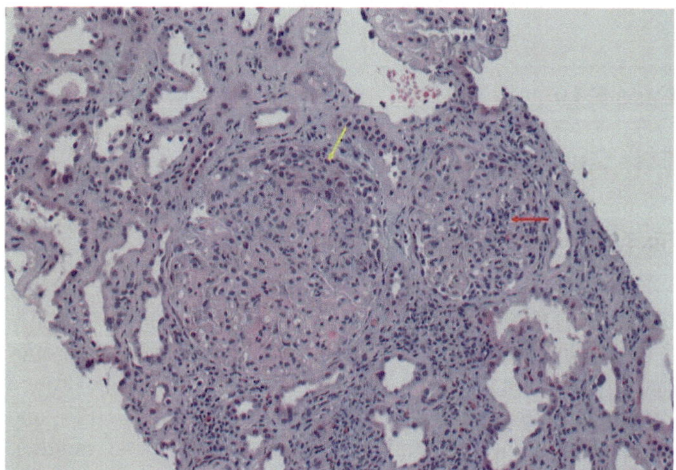

Fig. 5.23 Increased intracapillary and mesangial cellularity with PMNs (red arrow), and a small cellular crescent (yellow arrow). H&E, 20×

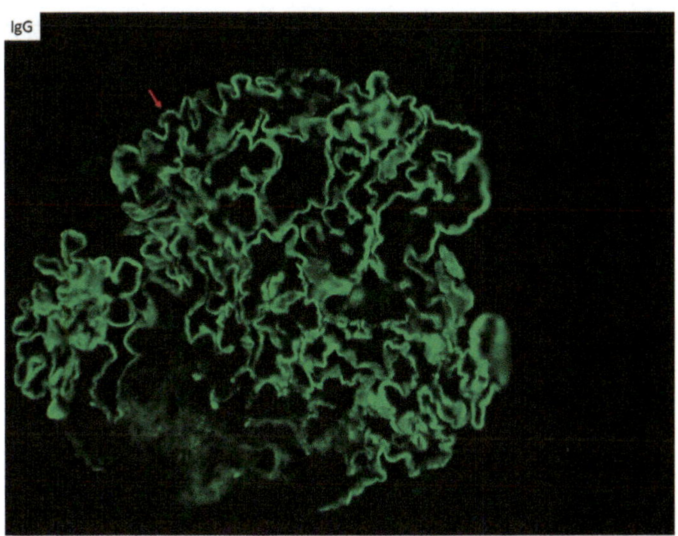

Fig. 5.24 IgG immunofluorescence granular staining in the capillary walls red arrow, IF, 40×

- Possibility of concurrent acute cellular rejection could not be ruled out based solely on histopathology and did not meet criteria per Banff (ptc1, t1).

Management Approach

Triggering Factors

Likely due to a combination of autoimmune activation and alloimmune response, driven by nonadherence and under-immunosuppression.

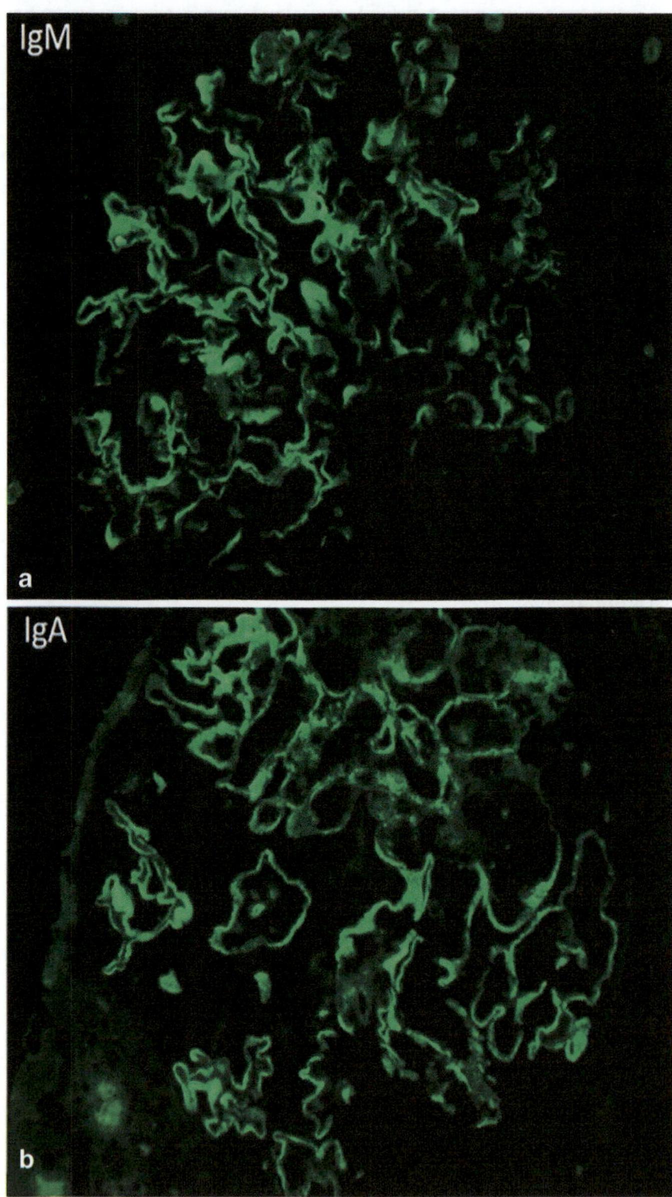

Fig. 5.25 Similar, granular staining on the capillary loop for: (**a**) IgM; (**b**) IgA; (**c**) C1q; (**d**) C3 by IF

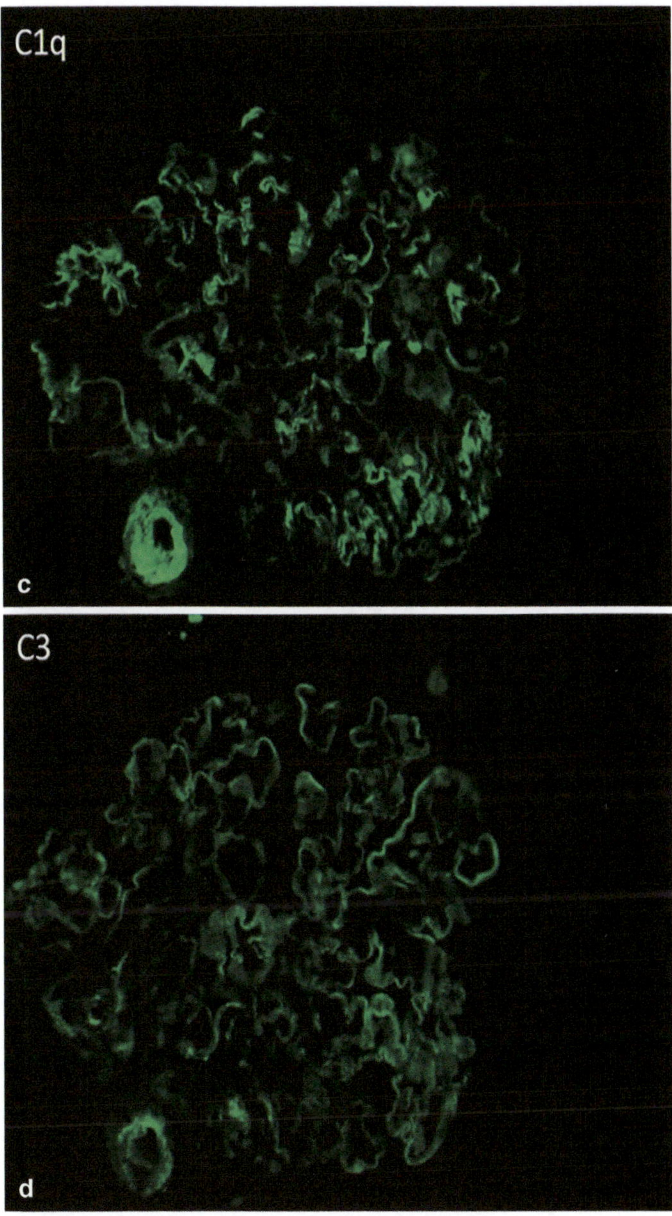

Fig. 5.25 (continued)

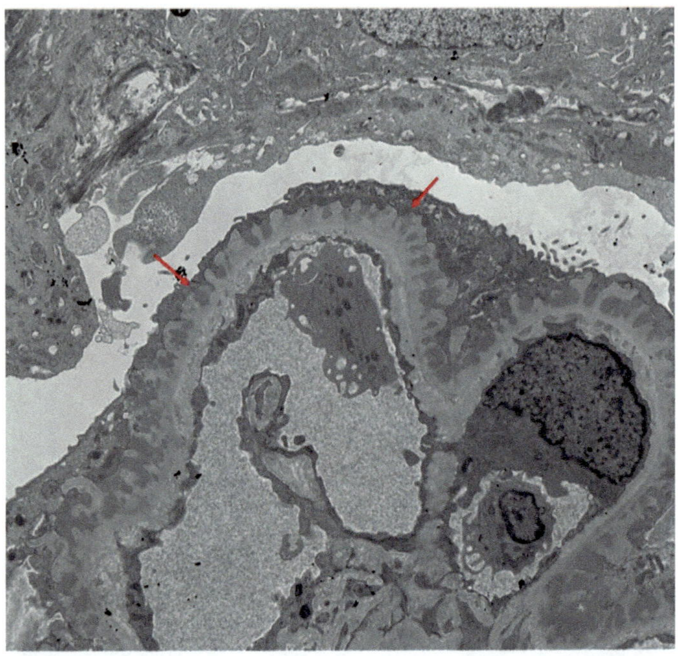

Fig. 5.26 Subepithelial electron dense deposits, red arrows. EM 6500×

Treatment

- Initiated pulse corticosteroids (Solu-Medrol).
- Switched from azathioprine to mycophenolate mofetil (MMF).

Follow-Up

Unfortunately, the patient progressed to graft failure and required initiation of dialysis.

Educational Insights

- De novo lupus nephritis post-kidney transplant is extremely rare, in contrast to the more common scenario of recurrent lupus nephritis in patients transplanted for SLE-related ESRD. And even recurrent is infrequent with large registry and cohort studies reporting rates of 1–10% and most cases being mild and subclinical due to the immunosuppressive environment following any transplant case.
- The American College of Rheumatology guideline notes that recurrence of lupus nephritis in the allograft is rare and typically mild, and does not discuss de novo SLE nephritis as a significant clinical entity after transplantation [18].
- In this case, nonadherence to immunosuppression likely led to both autoimmune reactivation and alloimmune injury, highlighting the importance of adherence in transplant recipients.
- The overlap of de novo autoimmune glomerulonephritis and rejection poses diagnostic and therapeutic challenges, especially when biopsy findings suggest possible coexisting pathology.

Pearl 5.10

De novo *SLE nephritis after kidney transplantation is exceedingly rare compared to recurrent SLE, FSGS, calcineurin inhibitor-associated nephropathy, or other viral-associated glomerular disease, all of which are more common and clinically significant causes of post-transplant glomerular pathology.*

Case 5.11

Case Study Summary

Patient: A 39-year-old male with end-stage renal disease (ESRD) secondary to diabetes mellitus.

Transplant course: He received a deceased donor kidney transplant (DDKT). Stable allograft function on traditional triple immunosuppression including CNI, MMF, and daily prednisone.

Clinical course: Two years post-transplant, he developed nephrotic-range proteinuria (5 g/g based on multiple random urine protein creatinine ratios) and microscopic hematuria. His infectious and autoimmune serology workup was negative, and his diabetes was well-controlled.

Diagnostic Workup

- Rejection workup: Negative by both histology and molecular diagnostics platforms (MMDx), undetectable donor-specific antibodies (DSA), and donor-derived cell-free DNA (dd-cfDNA).
- Viral and other serologies workup: negative for autoimmune, viral hepatitis, monoclonal gammopathy, or circulating cryoglobulins.
- Kidney biopsy revealed diffuse mesangial and endocapillary proliferative glomerulonephritis, consistent with membranoproliferative glomerulonephritis (MPGN), with dominant IgG, C3, and codominant C1q deposits with mesangial and subendothelial electron-dense deposits (full house staining pattern).

Diagnosis

De novo immune complex-mediated MPGN (Figs. 5.27, 5.28, and 5.29) with full-house immunofluorescence pattern (Fig. 5.28).

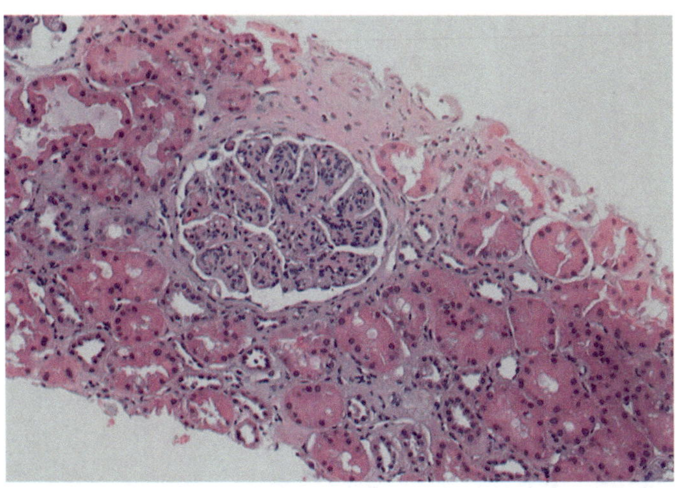

Fig. 5.27 MPGN injury pattern with increased endocapillary and mesangial cellularity with a lobular pattern, H&E, 20×

Management Approach

- Poor response to oral steroids prompted escalation in immunosuppression.
- Initiated rituximab to augment immunosuppression.

Follow-Up

- Six years post-diagnosis:
  - Partial glomerular disease remission (UPCR reduced to 1 g/g and remained stable).
  - Stable graft function at CKD stage 3a.

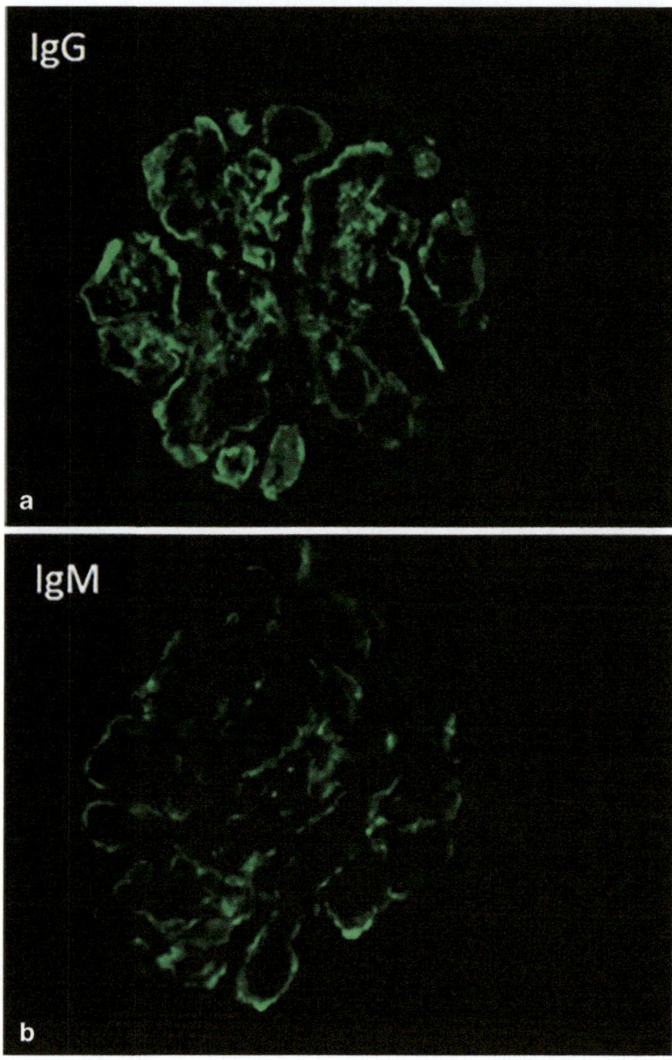

Fig. 5.28 IF "full house" staining in the capillary walls and mesangial areas. (**a**) IgG, (**b**) IgM, (**c**) IgA, (**d**) C1q, (**e**) C3

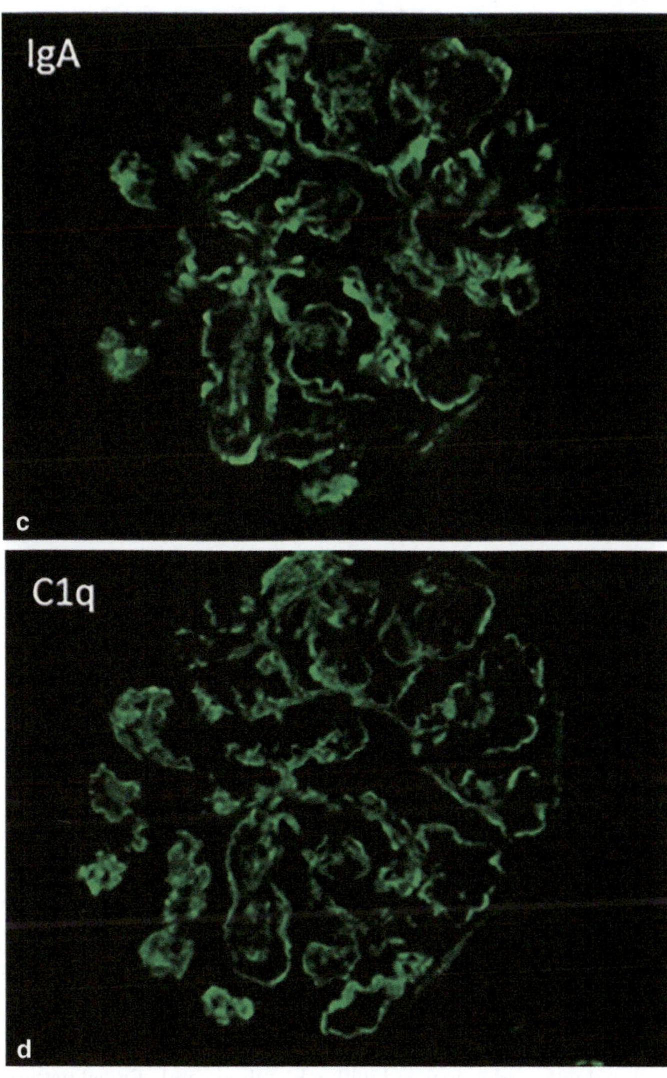

Fig. 5.28 (continued)

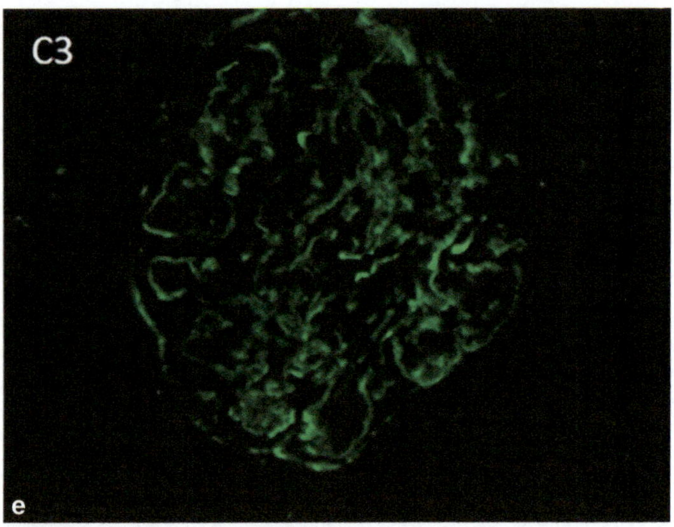

Fig. 5.28 (continued)

Educational Learning Points

- De novo immune complex–mediated glomerulonephritis, including MPGN diagnosis, is mainly based on immunofluorescence findings, and this could be related to different subtypes.
- Cases with mesangial and capillary complement deposits and lack of Ig deposition on immunofluorescence are classified as C3 glomerulopathy (either dense deposit disease or C3 GN). Cases with capillary and mesangial deposits of Igs are classified as Ig-mediated MPGN like in this case.
- Pathogenesis is poorly understood, de novo MPGN pattern of injury reported in autoimmune disease, HCV-positive patients, cryoglobulinemia, monoclonal gammopathy including myeloma, and associated with a histologic and clinical pattern of de novo thrombotic microangiopathy, a condition that may be triggered by rejection, CNI toxicity or viral infection [19].

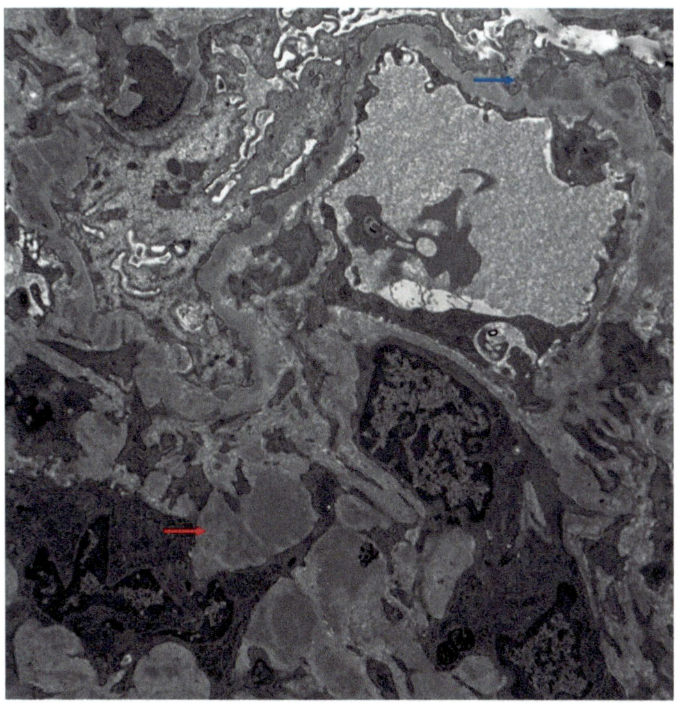

Fig. 5.29 Mesangial (red arrow) and subepithelial (blue arrow) electron dense deposits, EM 8000×

Pearl 5.11

De novo *immune complex-mediated glomerulonephritis post-transplant is classified by immunofluorescence patterns into C3 glomerulopathy (complement-only deposits) or Ig-mediated MPGN (immunoglobulin and complement deposits). Its causes are unclear but may involve autoimmune disease, infections, monoclonal gammopathy, or injury from rejection and drug toxicity.*

Case 5.12

Clinical Study Summary

Patient: A 66-year-old male with ESRD secondary to type 2 diabetes mellitus.

Transplant course: He received a deceased donor kidney transplant (DDKT) from an HCV NAT-positive donor. Post-transplant treatment included induction therapy with (ATG), steroids and direct-acting antiviral (DAA) therapy achieving sustained virologic response (SVR) for HCV. Prophylaxis with entecavir was initiated due to donor HBV core antibody positivity.

Clinical Course: Approximately 2 years post-transplant, the patient developed volume overload, nephrotic-range proteinuria (5 g/g based on multiple random urine protein creatinine ratios), microscopic hematuria, lower extremities rash, and acute kidney injury (creatinine raised from 1.0 to 1.6 mg/dL). This episode was preceded by a methicillin-sensitive *Staphylococcus aureus* (MSSA) psoas abscess.

Laboratory evaluation: Revealed positive type III cryoglobulinemia without detectable monoclonal proteins; serologies and donor-specific antibodies (DSA) were negative, and donor-derived cell-free DNA (dd-cfDNA) levels were not elevated. Skin biopsy confirmed cryoglobulinemic vasculitis presenting as purplish, flat rashes on the lower extremities and forearms.

Diagnosis

- Differential diagnosis included de novo IgA nephropathy versus IgA-dominant post-infectious glomerulonephritis (PIGN), in the light of the recent MSSA infection (Figs. 5.30, 5.31, and 5.32).
- The positive cryoglobulin test for cryoglobulinemia type 3 was noted; however, no definite organized substructure of the electron-dense deposits by the electron microscopy was identified.

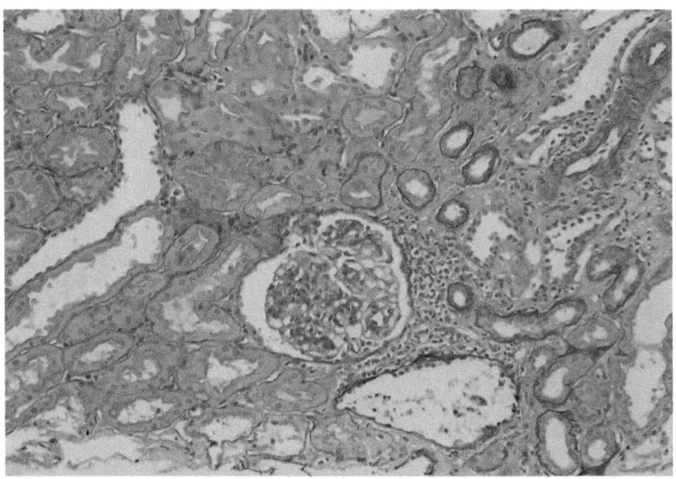

Fig. 5.30 Glomerulus with no significant capillary or mesangial increased cellularity. PAS, 20×

Management Approach

Triggering factors: The clinical presentation was likely triggered by MSSA infection and subsequent immune complex formation.

Treatment: Comprised antibiotics, steroids, angiotensin receptor blockers (ARB), and SGLT2 inhibitor therapy.

Follow-Up

- The patient demonstrated clinical improvement with antibiotic therapy and immunosuppression adjustments.

Educational Insights

- In transplant recipients, IgA-dominant PIGN is rare but clinically significant in kidney transplant recipients, with a variable prognosis including graft loss.

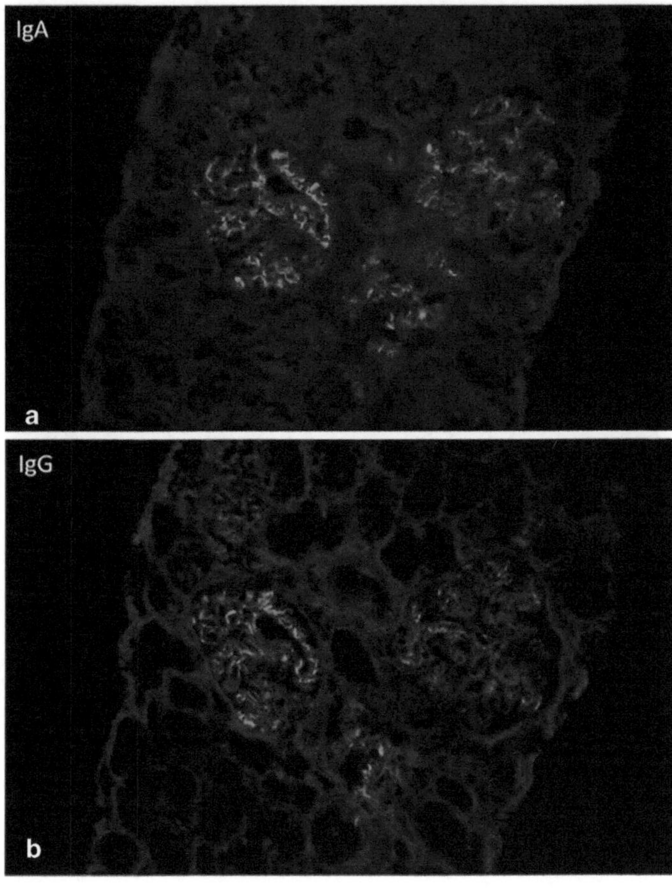

Fig. 5.31 (**a**) IgA 2/3 + mesangial granular staining by IF, (**b**) IgG 2+ mesangial granular staining by IF

- It is temporally associated with bacterial infection, most commonly following Staphylococcus or, less frequently, Gram-negative organisms [20, 21] and must be distinguished from de novo IgA nephropathy.

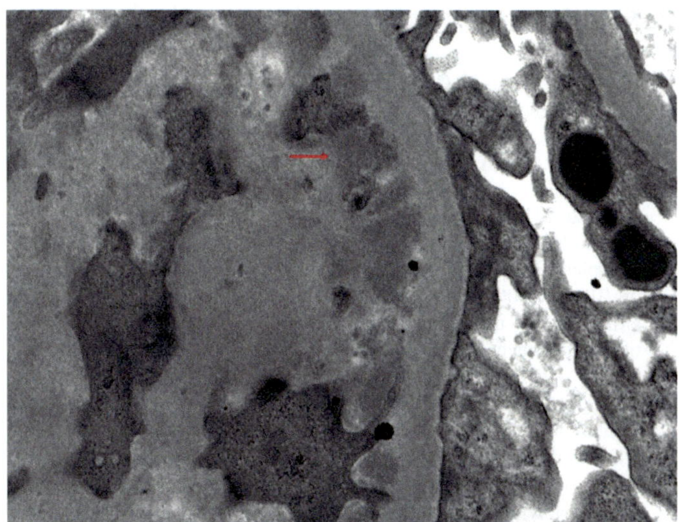

Fig. 5.32 Mesangial electron dense deposits (red arrow) EM 6000×

- Type III cryoglobulinemia are composed of mixed polyclonal IgG and IgM, may accompany autoimmune disorders or infections (bacterial or viral such as HCV), and could contribute to glomerular injury and systemic vasculitis.
- Early recognition and treatment of infection-related glomerulonephritis are critical to preserving graft function.

Pearl 5.12

IgA-dominant post-infectious glomerulonephritis, though rare in transplant recipients, can lead to significant graft dysfunction and must be distinguished from de novo *IgA nephropathy. Often triggered by bacterial infections like Staphylococcus, it may be accompanied by type 3 cryoglobulinemia, contributing to vasculitis and glomerular injury. Early diagnosis and infection-directed therapy are essential to preserving graft function.*

References

1. Medieral-Thomas N. Complement activation in IgA nephropathy. Semin Immunopathol. 2021;43(5):679–90. https://doi.org/10.1007/s00281-021-00882-9.
2. Ramsawak S. IgA nephropathy: update on pathogenesis and treatment. Cleve Clin J Med. 2025;92(6):373–83. https://doi.org/10.3949/ccjm.92a.24105.
3. Obermiller LE. Recurrent membranous glomerulonephritis in two renal transplants. Transplantation. 1985;40:100–2. https://doi.org/10.1097/00007890-198507000-00020.
4. Grupper A. Recurrent membranous nephropathy after kidney transplantation: treatment and long-term implications. Transplantation. 2016;100(12):2710–6. https://doi.org/10.1097/TP.0000000000001056.
5. Hullekes F. Recurrence of membranous nephropathy after kidney transplantation: a multicenter retrospective cohort study. Am J Transplant. 2024;24(6):1016–26. https://doi.org/10.1016/j.ajt.2024.01.036.
6. Kanai T. Predominant but silent C1q deposits in mesangium on transplanted kidneys – long-term observational study. BMC Nephrol. 2018;19(1):82. https://doi.org/10.1186/s12882-018-0874-9.
7. Said SM. C1q deposition in the renal allograft: a report of 24 cases. Mod Pathol. 2010;23(8):1080–8. https://doi.org/10.1038/modpathol.2010.92.
8. Sethi S. Mayo clinic/renal pathology society consensus report on pathologic classification, diagnosis, and reporting of GN. J Am Soc Nephrol. 2016;27(5):1278–87. https://doi.org/10.1681/ASN.2015060612.
9. Khanna A. Expression of TGF-beta and Fibrogenic genes in transplant recipients with tacrolimus and cyclosporine nephrotoxicity. Kidney Int. 2002;62(6):2257–63.
10. Eberhardt W. Activation of renal Profibrotic TGFβ controlled signaling cascades by calcineurin and mTOR inhibitors. Cell Signal. 2018;52:1–11. https://doi.org/10.1016/j.cellsig.2018.08.013.
11. Larsen C. Membranoproliferative glomerulonephritis with masked monotypic immunoglobulin deposits. Kidney Int. 2015;88(4):867–73. https://doi.org/10.1038/ki.2015.195.
12. Coyne BM. Ascertaining the mechanistic etiology of COVID-associated glomerulonephritis: a systematic review. Front Med. 2025;12:1568943. https://doi.org/10.3389/fmed.2025.1568943.
13. George JA. SARS-CoV-2 infection and the kidneys: an evolving picture. Adv Exp Med Biol. 2021;1327:107–18. https://doi.org/10.1007/978-3-030-71697-4_8.
14. Shetty AA. COVID-19-associated glomerular disease. J Am Soc Nephrol. 2021;32(1):33–40. https://doi.org/10.1681/ASN.2020060804.
15. Alhamad T. ACTH gel in resistant focal segmental Glomerulosclerosis after kidney transplantation. Transplantation. 2019;103(1):202.

16. Alasfar S. Rituximab and therapeutic plasma exchange in recurrent focal segmental Glomerulosclerosis Postkidney transplantation. Transplantation. 2018;102(3):e115.
17. Uffing A. Recurrence of FSGS after kidney transplantation in adults. CJASN. 2020;15(2):247–56. https://doi.org/10.2215/CJN.08970719.
18. Sammaritano LR. American College of Rheumatology (ACR) guideline for the screening, treatment, and management of lupus nephritis. Arthritis Rheumatol. 2024, 2025; https://doi.org/10.1002/art.43212.
19. Ponticelli C. De Novo glomerular diseases after renal transplantation. CJASN. 2014;9(8):1479–87. https://doi.org/10.2215/CJN.12571213.
20. Moroni G. Acute post-bacterial glomerulonephritis in renal transplant patients: description of three cases and review of the literature. Am J Transplant. 2004;4(1):132–6.
21. Basic-Jukic N. IgA-dominant extracapillary proliferative glomerulonephritis following Escherichia coli sepsis in a renal transplant recipient. Transpl Infect Dis. 2018;20(5):e12927. https://doi.org/10.1111/tid.12927.

Recurrent Post-transplant Glomerulonephritis

6

Ana Lia Castellanos

Case 6.1

Case Study Summary

The patient is a 46-year-old African American male with a history of end-stage renal disease (ESRD) secondary to idiopathic membranous nephropathy.

He underwent a deceased donor kidney transplant (DDKT), KDPI 11%, 3/6 HLA mismatch with a calculated panel-reactive antibody (cPRA) of 8%. Induction therapy included antithymocyte globulin (ATG), and maintenance regimen included tacrolimus, mycophenolate mofetil, and daily prednisone.

Post-transplant Clinical Course

Three weeks after transplant high nadir Serum creatinine of 2.5 and new onset proteinuria, spot urine protein-to-creatinine ratio (UPCR) of 1 g/g.

A. L. Castellanos (✉)
Division of Nephrology, Bone and Mineral Metabolism, University of Kentucky, Medical Center, Lexington, KY, USA
e-mail: AnaCastellanos@uky.edu

H. Fattah, V. Cornea (eds.), *Transplantation in Practice*,
https://doi.org/10.1007/978-3-032-15908-3_6

Negative workup including renal transplant ultrasound, donor-specific antibodies (DSA), and donor-derived cell-free DNA (dd-cfDNA). PLA2R antibody was undetectable one year prior to kidney transplantation.

Diagnosis

- Recurrent iMN, positive PLA2R ab as evident from (Figs. 6.1, 6.2, and 6.3).
- No evidence of acute cellular rejection (ACR) or antibody-mediated rejection (ABMR) on renal allograft biopsy.

Management Approach

No clear triggering factors identified, although no pre-kidney transplant PLA2R antibody was available and PLA2R antibody was negative 1 year prior to kidney transplantation.

Patient therapy included the addition of ARB therapy and rituximab.

Continued immunosuppressive regimen of tacrolimus, mycophenolate mofetil, and daily prednisone.

Follow-Up

There was no significant improvement of serum creatinine but improvement of proteinuria to a UPCR below 0.2 g/g.

Educational Insights

- In patients with known iMN who are being evaluated for kidney transplantation, it is very important to determine the type of MN present in the native kidney biopsy and specifically if MN is related to autoantibodies to the phospholipase A2 receptor (PLA2R) [2, 3].

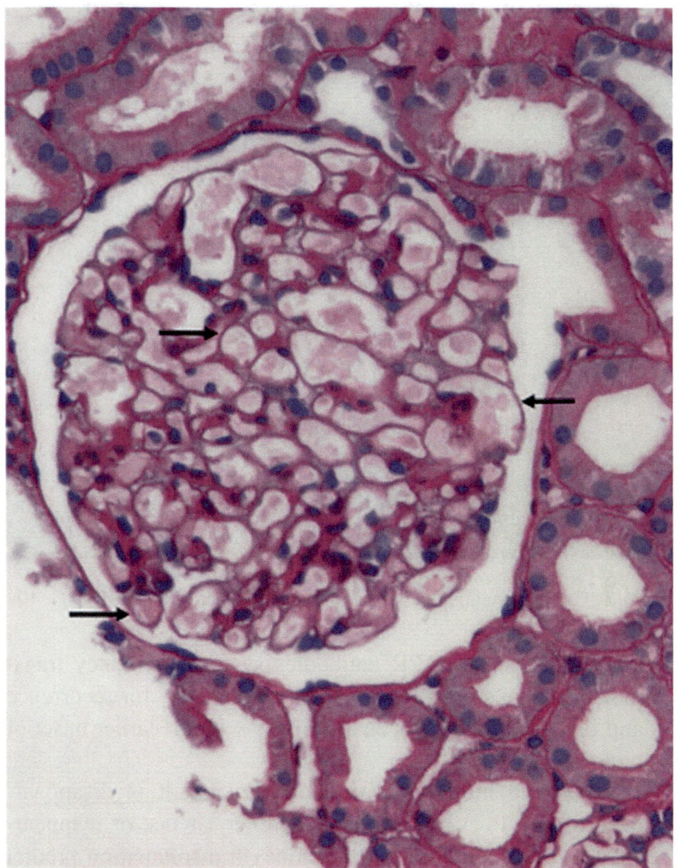

Fig. 6.1 Capillaries with thick and rigid wall (black arrows). PAS, 20×

- In patients with known PLA2R-associated MN, it is important to test for circulating anti-PLA2R antibodies as part of the initial workup for kidney transplantation to determine and assess the risk of recurrence [2].
- Reported incidence of recurrent MN in Kidney transplant recipients ranges between 10 and 45%. Rapid recurrence of MN after kidney transplantation suggests the potential presence of a circulatory autoantibody to the M-type PLA2R [1, 3].

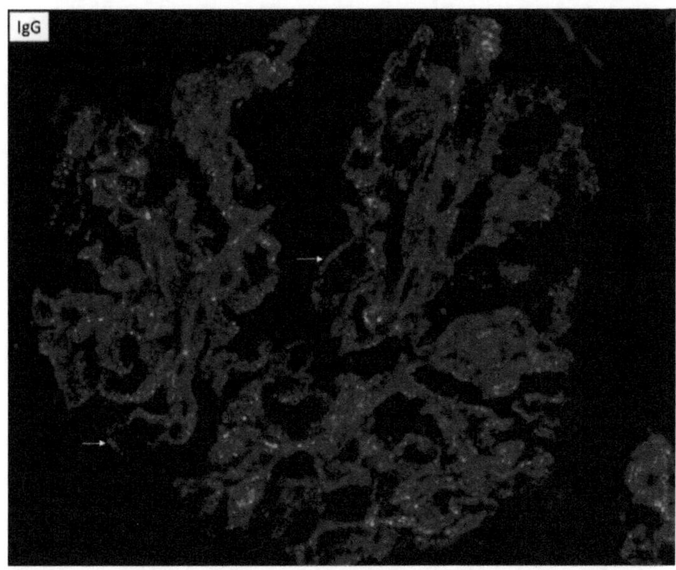

Fig. 6.2 Granular staining in the capillary walls (white arrows), IF IgG, 40×

- Circulating anti-PLA2R antibodies at or after kidney transplantation have been identified as a risk factor for recurrence and higher titers have been associated with an earlier onset of recurrence [3, 4].
- Maintenance immunosuppression may result in disappearance of anti-PLA2R antibodies and persistence or reappearance of these antibodies after kidney transplantation predict worse clinical course with increasing and persistent proteinuria [3, 4].
- Treatment will vary based on disease severity, including continued immunosuppression, addition of ACEI/ARB, SGLT2 Inhibitors and the use of Rituximab for moderate to severe disease.

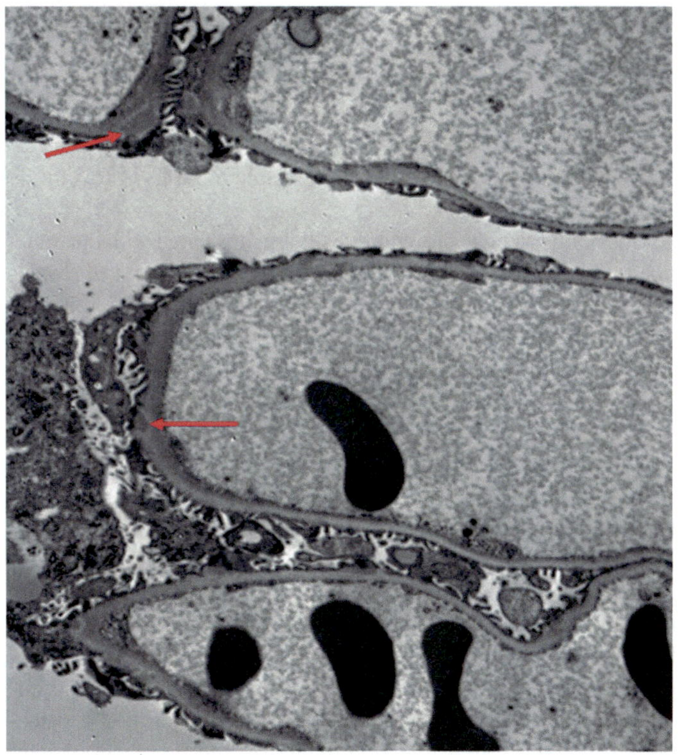

Fig. 6.3 Subepithelial electron-dense deposits (red arrows), EM, 6000× (red arrows)

Pearl 6.1

Idiopathic MN is an autoimmune disease, which can occur any time after kidney transplantation, literature suggests higher recurrence in under immunosuppressed patients or those patients with positive PLA2R ab prior to transplantation. Proteinuria, a marker of disease remission can lag behind immunologic remission.

Case 6.2

Case Study Summary

The patient is a 46-year-old Caucasian female with a history of chronic kidney disease (CKD) stage 5, due to biopsy-proven IgA nephropathy.

She underwent a pre-emptive living unrelated kidney transplant (LUKT), 5/6 HLA mismatch, with a calculated panel-reactive antibody (cPRA) of 0%. Induction therapy included antithymocyte globulin (ATG), maintenance regimen included tacrolimus, mycophenolate mofetil, and daily prednisone.

Post-transplant Clinical Course

Her course was complicated by rising serum creatinine and elevated donor-derived cell free DNA (dd-cfDNA) and biopsy-proven TCMR 2A and subclinical IgA pattern on her biopsy, with no clinical active urine sediment at the time. She was treated with IV Solu-Medrol pulse and prednisone recycle and antithymocyte globulin (ATG) with improvement of her renal function and dd-cfDNA. Repeat renal allograft biopsy showed resolution of rejection. Three years after rejection diagnosis and treatment, patient developed microscopic hematuria and sub-nephrotic range proteinuria, prompting repeat renal allograft biopsy and repeat biopsy with clear evidence of IgA nephropathy.

Diagnosis

- Recurrent IgA nephropathy seen under LM and IF in (Figs. 6.4, 6.5, and 6.6).
- No evidence of ACR or antibody-mediated rejection (ABMR) on renal allograft biopsy.

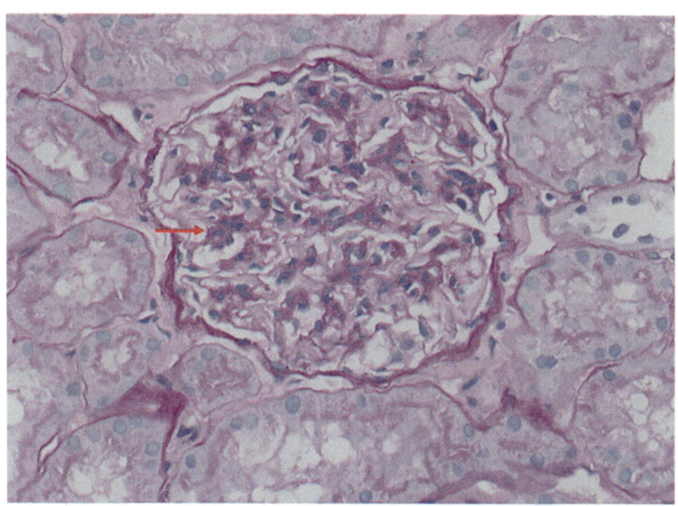

Fig. 6.4 Slightly increased mesangial cellularity (red arrow), PAS stain, 40×

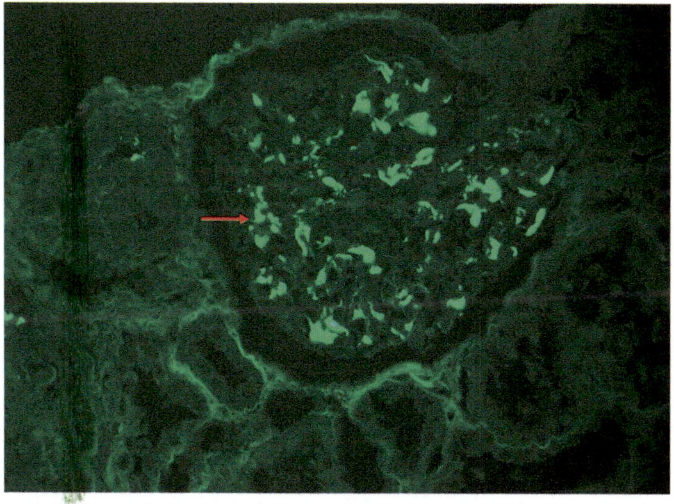

Fig. 6.5 2–3+ granular mesangial staining for IgA (red arrow). Immunofluorescence microscopy

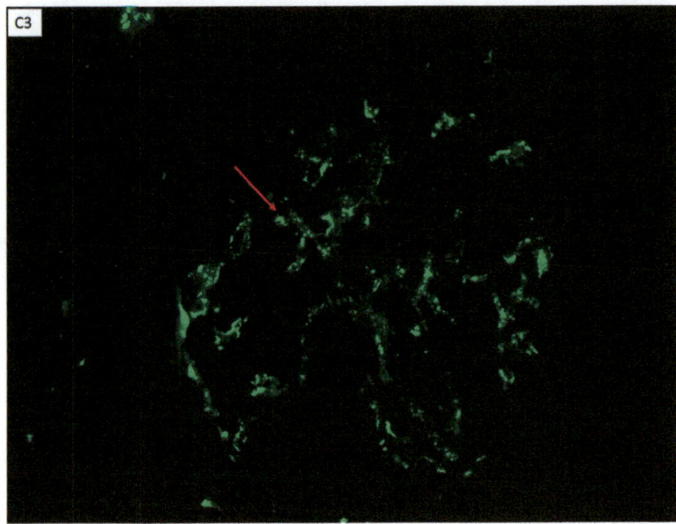

Fig. 6.6 C3 3+ granular mesangial staining (red arrow). Immunofluorescence

Management Approach

No clear triggering factors were identified.

Patient therapy included ARB therapy and prednisone that due to significant side effects was later changed to Budesonide, which she took for 9 months.

Continued immunosuppressive regimen of tacrolimus, mycophenolate mofetil, and daily prednisone.

Follow-Up

She developed complete remission with stable allograft function 5 years after kidney transplant and bland urinalysis on last check.

Educational Insights

- Incidence of recurrence of IgAN in the transplanted kidney varies in the literature, based on the time or indication for biopsy. The main predictor for recurrence is longer time after transplantation [5].
- Histologic recurrence is common and incidence ranges between 20% and 60% [5].
- The Oxford classification of IgAN has prognostic value in kidney transplant recipients with recurrent IgAN.
- Early glucocorticoid withdrawal after kidney transplantation has been associated with increased risk of recurrence of IgAN and continued use of glucocorticoids post-kidney transplant has been associated with decreased risk of recurrence [6].
- Treatment of recurrent IgAN will vary based on disease activity and presentation. The use of ACEI/ARB is recommended. For patients with more aggressive disease, including rising serum creatinine and significant proteinuria, high-dose glucocorticoids are recommended.
- Budesonide has been reported to cause significant proteinuria reduction in transplanted patients with less adverse events when compared to high-dose glucocorticoid therapy [7].

Pearl 6.2

Recurrence of IgA nephropathy is common after kidney transplantation with an incidence of 20–30% and up to 60% on protocol or surveillance biopsies.

Case 6.3

Case Study Summary

The patient is a 31-year-old Caucasian male with a history of end-stage renal disease (ESRD) secondary to focal segmental glomerulosclerosis (FSGS). Had a deceased donor kidney transplant (DDKT) that failed 10 years later due to recurrent FSGS. He received a second DDKT, KDPI 17%, and calculated panel-reactive antibody (cPRA) of 0%. Induction therapy included anti-thymocyte globulin (ATG), maintenance regimen included tacrolimus, mycophenolate mofetil, and prednisone.

Post-transplant Clinical Course

One-year post Kidney transplantation, patient developed nephrotic syndrome with a UPCR of 6.5 g/g, no microscopic hematuria and no change in serum creatinine.

Negative workup including renal transplant ultrasound, DSA, and donor-derived cell-free DNA (dd-cfDNA).

Diagnosis

- Recurrent idiopathic FSGS in second kidney transplant, features of segmental scars under LM (Fig. 6.7) and complete foot process effacement under EM (Fig. 6.8).
- No evidence of ACR or antibody-mediated rejection (ABMR) on renal allograft biopsy.

Management Approach

Some of the triggering factors identified include his younger age at disease onset, rapid progression of his initial disease, and history of recurrence in his previous allograft.

Patient therapy included continued immunosuppressive regimen of tacrolimus, mycophenolate mofetil and prednisone as well as ARB and SGLT2 inhibitor, patient later needed escalation of treatment due to inadequate response these advanced treatment included plasma exchange, and obinutuzumab.

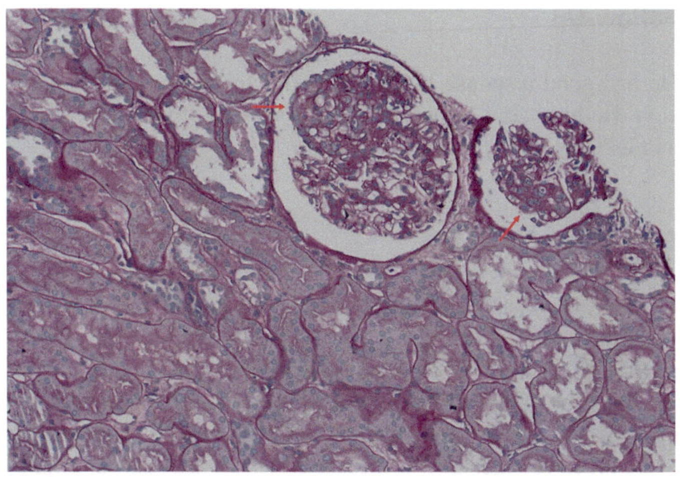

Fig. 6.7 Segmental glomerular scar, FSGS (red arrows). PAS, 20×

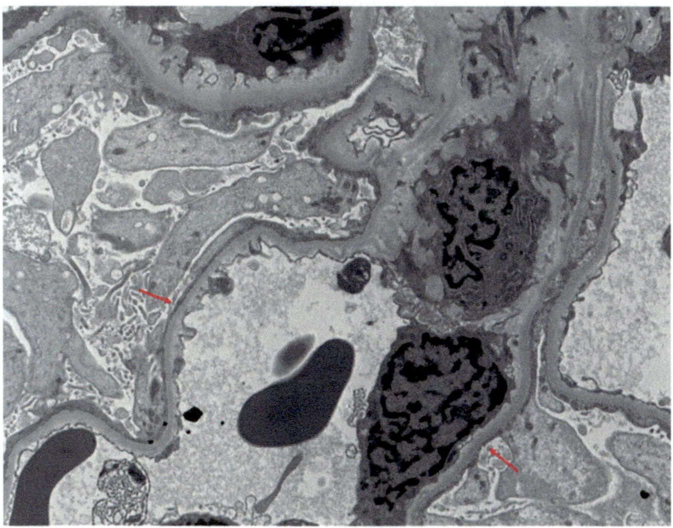

Fig. 6.8 Marked effacement of foot processes (red arrows). EM, 1200×

Follow-Up

He had good response to therapy and achieved complete remission. He has stable allograft function 4 years after his diagnosis and UPCR of 0.3 g/g.

Educational Insights

- FSGS is a histologic pattern of injury in the kidney with many different etiologies.
- Primary FSGS may recur in the kidney allograft and all efforts should be made to identify this prior to transplantation.
- Risk factors for recurrence of FSGS post transplantation include: younger age at disease onset, Caucasian, rapid progression of initial disease, lower BMI at time of transplantation, and history of recurrence in a prior allograft [8].
- Post-transplant surveillance is important to identify recurrence and initiate treatment promptly [8].
- Optimal therapy may vary between transplant centers, timing of recurrence, and aggressiveness of disease. Plasmapheresis and rituximab alone or in combination with plasmapheresis are main stage of treatment. The use of ACEI/ARB and SGLT-2 inhibitors is also recommended [8, 9].

Pearl 6.3

Recurrent primary FSGS is common after kidney transplantation, and higher recurrence rates can occur with subsequent kidney transplants. Surveillance is important and treatment should be initiated early in efforts to achieve partial or complete remission with associated better long-term outcomes.

Case 6.4

Case Study Summary

The patient is a 55-year old Caucasian female with a history of end-stage renal disease (ESRD) secondary to focal segmental glomerulosclerosis (FSGS). She has a history of prior living donor kidney transplant (LDKT) that failed due to early recurrent FSGS. She received a second deceased donor kidney transplant (DDKT) complicated by early onset proteinuria within the first week of transplant.

She received empirical treatment for recurrent FSGS achieving partial remission. One-year post-kidney transplantation, a renal allograft biopsy showed persistent moderate foot process effacement on electron microscopy, minimal interstitial fibrosis, and tubular atrophy, and there was no evidence of rejection.

Post-transplant Clinical Course

First week post-kidney transplantation, she developed proteinuria with a spot urine protein-to-creatinine ratio (UPCR) of 2.4 g/g. She received empirical treatment for recurrent FSGS achieving partial remission and UPCR of 1.4 g/g. One-year post-KT, her renal function remained stable, UPCR of 0.6 g/g. Renal allograft biopsy with minimal interstitial fibrosis and tubular atrophy and persistent moderate foot process effacement on electron microscopy.

Diagnosis

- Early recurrent FSGS in second kidney transplant, EM findings of foot process effacement (Fig. 6.9).
- No evidence of ACR or antibody-mediated rejection (ABMR) on renal allograft biopsy.

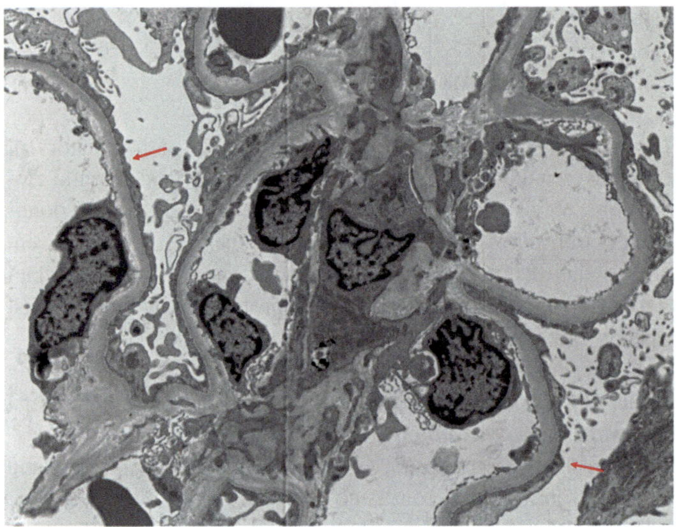

Fig. 6.9 Marked foot process effacement(red arrows). EM, 1200×

Management Approach

The main triggering factor in this patient was the history of early recurrence of FSGS after her first kidney transplant.

Continued immunosuppressive regimen of tacrolimus, mycophenolate mofetil, and prednisone. She was placed on ARB therapy, and due to persistent proteinuria and FSGS features on repeat biopsy a trial of LDL apheresis and finerenone was introduced later.

Follow-Up

Patient achieved partial remission with improvement of proteinuria of greater that 50%, UPCR of 0.6 g/g. She continues to have stable renal function (serum creatinine of 0.7) and non-nephrotic range proteinuria 5 years post-kidney transplant (kidney transplant number two).

Educational Insights

- Recurrence of FSGS post-transplantation can lead to graft loss. Close monitoring of recurrence is important and rapid implementation of treatment is vital in efforts to achieve complete or partial remission and improve outcomes [10].
- Low density lipoprotein apheresis (LDL-A) has shown promise in the treatment of nephrotic syndrome and FSGS. This procedure removes lipoproteins that contain apolipoprotein-B from the blood, with reduction in oxidized LDL and associated inflammatory cytokines and perhaps improves responsiveness to standard immunosuppression [11]
- Data is limited on the benefits of prophylactic measures to prevent recurrence of FSGS in the kidney allograft and it is not recommended [12].
- Despite the complete remission goal for nephrotic range, proteinuria yields the most favorable long-term prognosis; there is increasing body of evidence demonstrating that both complete and partial remission of proteinuria are independently associated with better renal survival and slower progression to ESRD compared to persistent proteinuria.

Pearl 6.4

Achieving partial or complete remission has been associated with better long-term outcomes in patients with recurrent FSGS after kidney transplantation. Treatment with LDL pheresis has some documented benefits in this patient population.

Case 6.5

Case Study Summary

The patient is a 41-year old Caucasian male with a history of end-stage renal disease (ESRD) of unknown etiology.

He underwent a living unrelated kidney transplant (LUKT), calculated panel-reactive antibody (cPRA) of 32% and 2/6 antigen match. Induction therapy included antithymocyte globulin (ATG); maintenance regimen included tacrolimus, mycophenolate mofetil, and daily prednisone.

Post-transplant Clinical Course

Eight years post-kidney transplantation patient developed new onset nephrotic syndrome with spot urine protein-to-creatinine ratio (UPCR) 10 g/g, microscopic hematuria, and rising serum creatinine.

He had negative workup including renal transplant ultrasound, DSA, and donor-derived cell-free DNA (dd-cfDNA). Immunologic work up was unrevealing.

Diagnosis

- De Novo versus Recurrent IgA Nephropathy with cellular crescents, MEST 3(M0, E1, S1, T1) (Figs. 6.10, 6.11, and 6.12).
- No evidence of ACR or antibody-mediated rejection (ABMR) on renal allograft biopsy.

Management Approach

No clear triggering factors were identified.

Patient therapy included IV/oral steroids, ARB and SGLT2 inhibitors.

Continued immunosuppressive regimen of tacrolimus, mycophenolate mofetil, and prednisone.

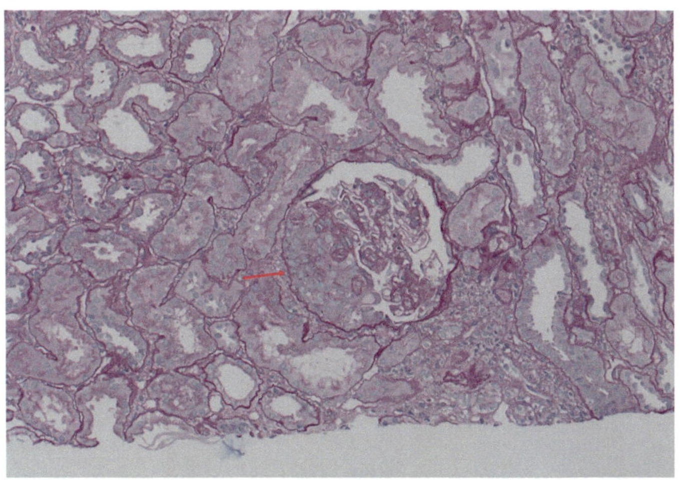

Fig. 6.10 Cellular crescent (red arrow). PAS, 20×

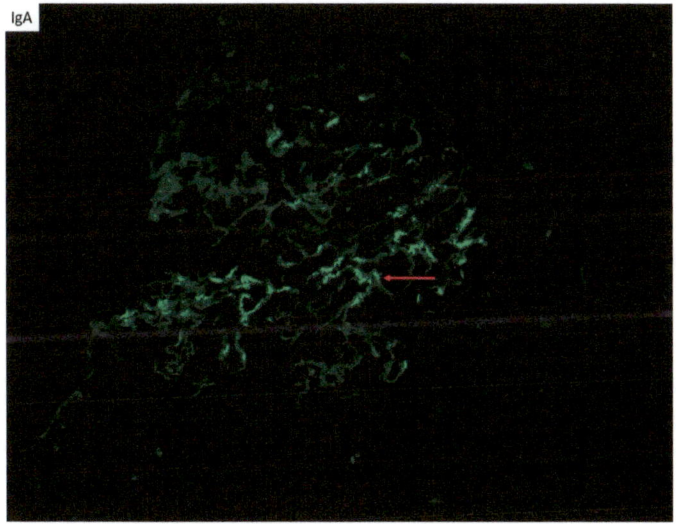

Fig. 6.11 Mesangial IgA-positive staining, Immune complex deposits (red arrow). IgA Immunofluorescence, 40×

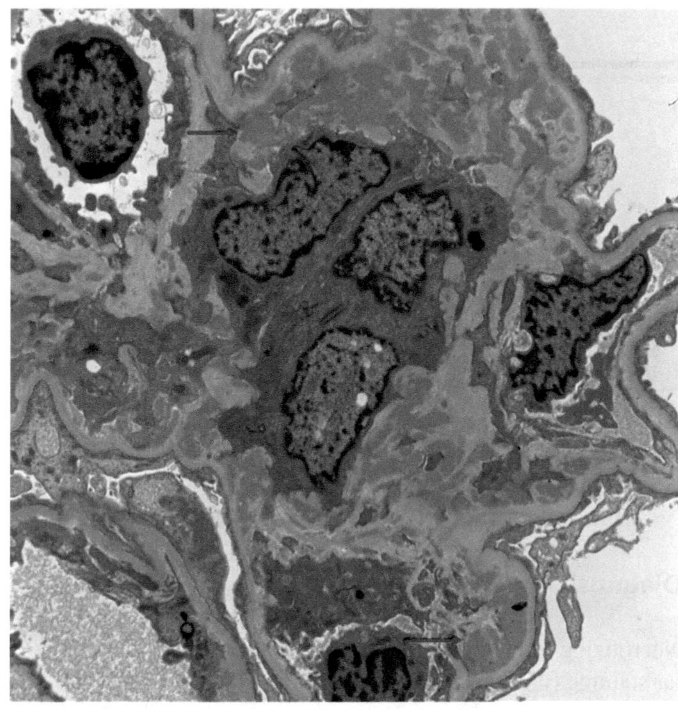

Fig. 6.12 Mesangial electron dense deposits (red arrows). EM, 6500×

Follow-Up

Patient was followed closely, and a repeat renal allograft biopsy 2 years later revealed persistent IgA nephropathy with advanced chronicity. Nephrotic syndrome had resolved, UPCR down to 0.6 g/g, and eGFR which had dropped 10 ml/min/1.73 m2 at the time of diagnosis has remained stable at 5-year follow-up with fluctuating eGFR between 30 and 32 ml/min/1.73 m^2.

Educational Insights

- Clinical and histologic risk factors have been identified in IgA nephropathy and can be used to risk stratify patients. Worse prognosis has been associated with presence of proteinuria (higher risk of progression in patients with UPCR >1 g/g), presence of hypertension, reduced eGFR at the time of diagnosis, and pathologic findings which add accuracy of prognosis over any clinical feature alone [13].
- The Oxford classification score (MEST-C score) was revised and is used to score kidney biopsies based on mesangial hypercellularity (M), endocapillary hypercellularity (E), segmental sclerosis (S), tubular atrophy/interstitial fibrosis (T), and crescents (C) [13].
- M, S, T, and C lesions of the classification independently predict the loss of eGFR and are associated with poor renal survival. T lesion is the strongest predictor of ESRD [13].
- The presence of crescents, cellular or fibrocellular, predicts poor renal outcomes. The addition of crescent scores, C1 (crescents in <25% of glomeruli) versus C0 (No crescents) versus C2 (crescents in >25% of glomeruli) can identify patients with poor renal outcome and response to therapy [14].

Pearl 6.5

The presence of any cellular or fibrocellular crescent is independently associated with worse prognosis in IgA Nephropathy. The Oxford classification has now added criteria for crescents, C0 (no crescents), C1 (less than 25% of glomeruli with crescents), and C2 (greater than 25% of glomeruli with crescents).

Case 6.6

Case Study Summary

The patient is a 33-year old African American Female with a history of end-stage renal disease (ESRD) secondary to SLE and SLE nephritis.

She underwent a deceased donor kidney transplant (DDKT), KDPI 9%, 4/6 HLA mismatch. Induction therapy included alemtuzumab, and steroids, maintenance regimen included tacrolimus, mycophenolate mofetil and prednisone.

Post-transplant Clinical Course

Patient with complicated post-operative course due to history of noncompliance, high intra-patient variability of tacrolimus (TacIPV), and unplanned pregnancy, prompting discontinuation of mycophenolate mofetil and starting azathioprine therapy. She was lost to follow-up and presented 5 years post-kidney transplant with acute on chronic kidney injury, serum creatinine of 3.4 from previous baseline of 1.4, microscopic hematuria with 100 RBC's, and proteinuria with UPCR of 5 g/g.

Renal transplant ultrasound, DSA and donor-derived cell-free DNA (dd-cfDNA) were unrevealing. Complement levels including C3 and C4 were normal. ANA and dsDNA were detected at low titers.

Diagnosis

- Recurrent lupus nephritis class 4 (diffuse proliferative), class 5 (membranous) with activity index of 6/24 and chronicity index of 8/12. Various slides to show pathologic evidence of recurrent LN (Figs. 6.13, 6.14, 6.15, and 6.16).
- No evidence of ACR or antibody-mediated rejection (ABMR) on renal allograft biopsy.

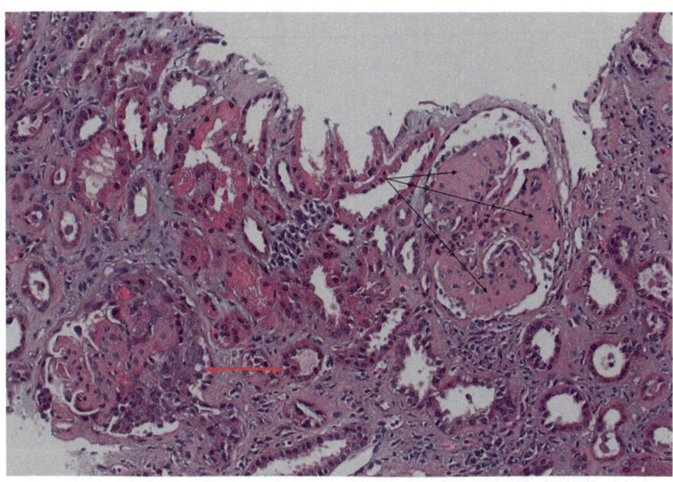

Fig. 6.13 Cellular crescent (red arrow), glomerular mesangial sclerosis (black arrows), H&E, 20×

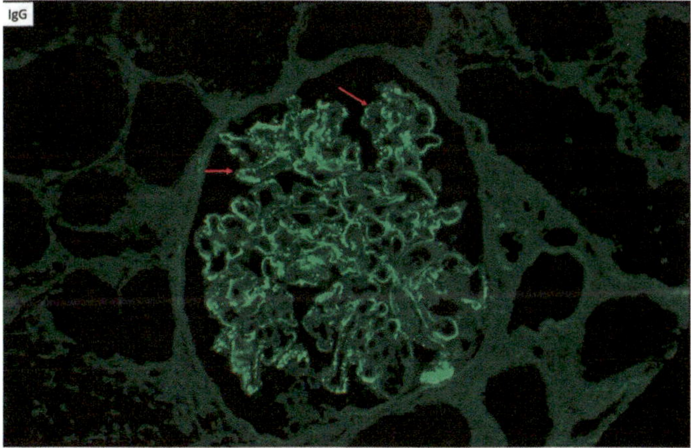

Fig. 6.14 IgG, 2–3+ granular staining in the capillary walls (red arrows), Immunofluorescence, 40×

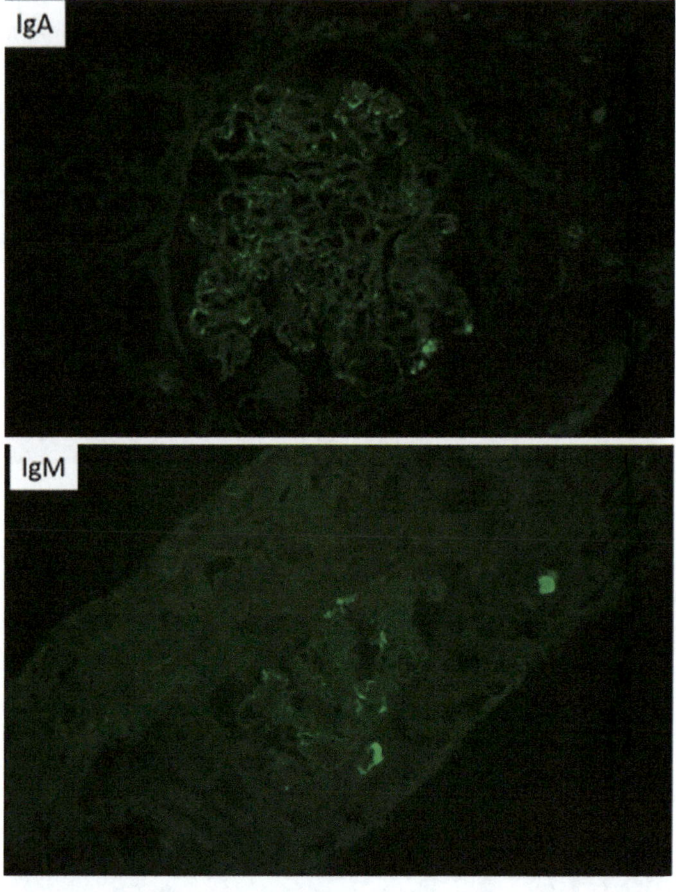

Fig. 6.15 IgA, IgM, C1q, C3, granular staining in the capillary walls. Full house immunofluorescence, 40×

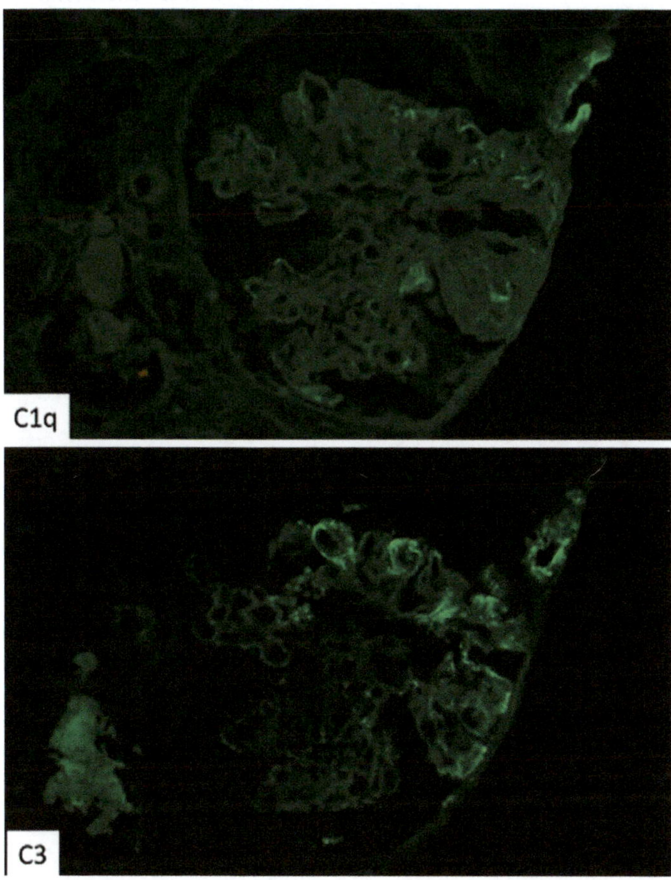

Fig. 6.15 (continued)

Management Approach

Main triggering factors identified were patient's young age, history of noncompliance both with medical appointments and medical therapy, and unplanned pregnancy.

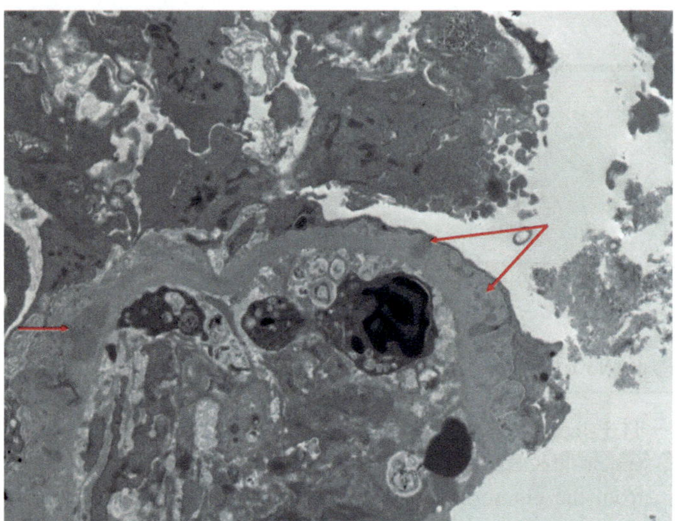

Fig. 6.16 Electron dense deposits in the subepithelial and intramembranous areas (red arrows) EM, 1200×

Upon diagnosis she was switched back to mycophenolate mofetil, azathioprine was discontinued. Compliance with immunosuppression was encouraged including continued immunosuppressive regimen of tacrolimus and prednisone.

Follow-Up

Due to high chronicity index, patient's kidney function continued to deteriorate. She had progressive renal dysfunction and allograft subsequently failed. She is now on renal replacement therapy in the forms of hemodialysis.

Educational Insights

- Lupus nephritis is a common and serious manifestation of lupus erythematosus. Achieving disease quiescence for at least

6 months, both serologically and clinically, is important prior to kidney transplantation [15].

- Compare to dialysis alone, patients with SLE nephritis who undergo kidney transplantation experience significantly improved prognosis and survival rates [15].
- Lupus nephritis recurrence following kidney transplantation varies across studies, but overall recurrence rate has been reported to be between 2% and 8% [15].
- Azathioprine has been found to increase disease relapse as maintenance therapy compared to mycophenolate mofetil [16].

Pearl 6.6

Relapse of lupus nephritis in the allograft is uncommon and if seen is usually in the setting of insufficient immune control or under immunosuppression. Serologic markers are unreliable predictors of relapse. Azathioprine has been associated with a higher rate of recurrence when compared to mycophenolate mofetil.

Case 6.7

Sravanthi Paluri

Case Study Summary

32-year-old white female with history of end-stage renal disease secondary to C3 glomerulonephritis (C3GN), gradual CKD progression, received brief period of Immunosuppression prior to undergoing living unrelated kidney transplant 7 years from diagnosis of C3GN. cPRA 16%, HLA 5/6 mismatch, and received thymoglobulin induction.

Post-transplant Clinical Course

- 6 months post-transplant, she had elevation in creatinine, urinalysis with mild protein, RBC, and WBC; cell-free DNA obtained was not elevated, but DSA were positive for class 2 Antibodies 2000–3000 MFI. Urine protein creatinine ratio was 0.4 g/g; complement levels c3 and c4 were low.
- C3 nephritic factor, factor H antibody, and factor B antibody tested were negative.
- She also had genetic testing for complement gene mutations which did not reveal any known pathogenic variants.
- Patient underwent renal allograft biopsy.

Diagnosis

Light microscopy—Recurrent C3GN. No evidence of acute cellular rejection. MPGN features on (Figs. 6.17 and 6.18).

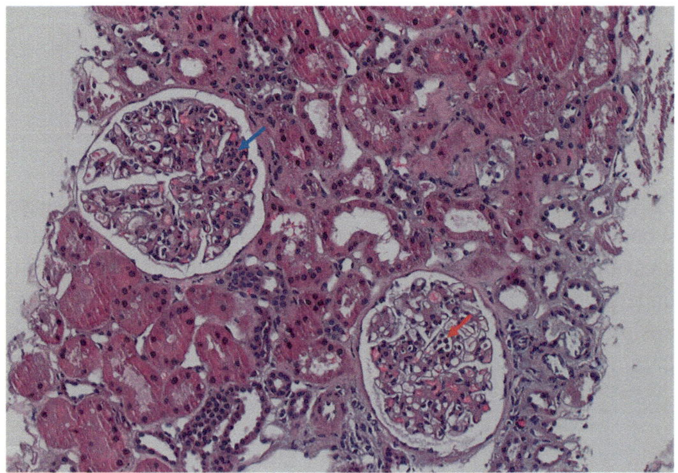

Fig. 6.17 Increased endocapillary (red arrow) and mesangial cellularity (blue arrow), H&E, 20×

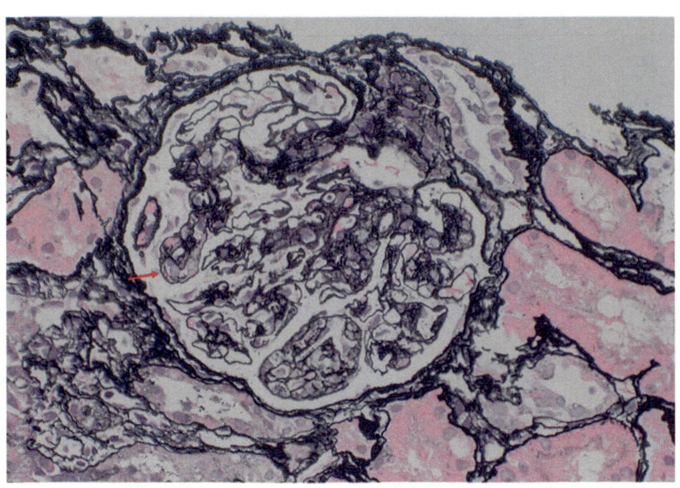

Fig. 6.18 GBM double contours (red arrow), Jones silver stain, 40×

Immunofluorescence microscopy—mesangial granular c3 staining (Fig. 6.19).

Electron microscopy—predominantly mesangial electron dense deposits in the glomeruli (Fig. 6.20)

Management Approach

Factors which likely contributed to development of recurrence:

- Subclinical antibody-mediated endothelial activation may worsen complement-mediated damage.

Treatment

Treatment with iptacopan a proximal complement inhibitor that binds factor B was considered, but patient was admitted with pyelonephritis.

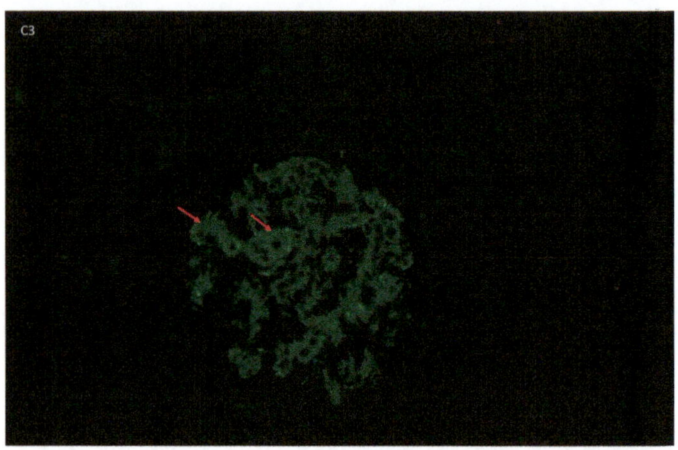

Fig. 6.19 Immunofluorescence: C3, granular mesangial staining, 40×

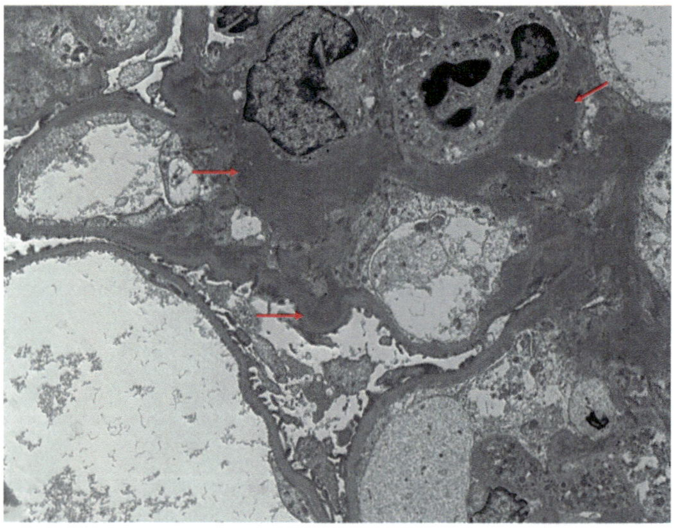

Fig. 6.20 Electron dense mesangial deposits (red arrows), 1200×

Patient received maximal immunosuppression for positive donor-specific antibodies and anti-proteinuria drugs—ACE inhibitors.

Follow-Up

- Stable graft function approaching 2 years post-transplant, proteinuria in remission and persistent urinary sediment and DSA.

Educational Insights

- This patient's native disease C3GN (with TMA on histology) was diagnosed in the setting of pregnancy that most likely had acquired (auto-antibodies) alternative complement pathway dysregulation. These abnormalities often remain after transplantation because they are constitutional and poorly influenced by the immunosuppression. [17]
- Challenges to the diagnosis of recurrent diseases are numerous, one of them being difficulties in differentiating recurrent disease from other causes of renal damage such as drug toxicity and chronic rejection [17, 18].
- The risk factors for recurrence and graft loss for C3GN are not well-defined. The broadest study on C3GN outcomes after recurrence by Zand et al. was unable to find any risk factor for recurrence [17].
- Post-transplant conditions that may cause endothelial insult include ischemia-reperfusion injury, infections, and immunosuppressive drugs. All of these factors could act as triggers to activate the AP in predisposed patients [17, 19]

Pearl 6.7

C3 glomerulonephritis represents a systemic disorder of alternative complement pathway dysregulation rather than a primary renal disease, and because the underlying defect persists after transplantation, recurrence in the allograft is very common.

Note: This chapter was authored by Dr. Ana Lia Castellanos and Dr. Sravanthi Paluri. It has been reviewed and edited by Dr. Hasan Fattah, the principal author, to maintain consistency with the rest of the book.

References

1. Dabade TS, Grande JP, Norby SM, et al. Recurrent idiopathic membranous nephropathy after kidney transplantation: a surveillance biopsy study. Am J Transplant. 2008;8:1318.
2. Stahl R, Hoxha E, Fechner K. PLA2R autoantibodies and recurrent membranous nephropathy after transplantation. N Engl J Med. 2010;363:496.
3. Quintana LF, Blasco M, Seras M, et al. Antiphospholipase A2 receptor antibody levels predict the risk of posttransplantation recurrence of membranous nephropathy. Transplantation. 2015;99:1709.
4. Hullekes F, Uffing A, et al. Recurrence of membranous nephropathy after kidney transplantation: a multicenter retrospective cohort study. Am J Transplant. 2024;24:1016–26.
5. Wyld M, Chadban S. Recurrent IgA nephropathy after kidney transplantation. Transplantation. 2016;100(9):1827–32.
6. Leeaphorn N, Garg N, Khankin EV, et al. Recurrence of IgA nephropathy after kidney transplantation in steroid continuation versus early steroid-withdrawal regimens: a retrospective analysis of the UNOS/OPTN database. Transplant Int. 2018;31:175.
7. Lopez-Martinez M, Soler MJ, et al. Enteric budesonide in transplant and native IgA nephropathy: real-world clinical practice. Transpl Int. 2022;35:10693.
8. Dantal J, Baatard R, Hourmant M, et al. Recurrent nephrotic syndrome following renal transplantation in patients with focal glomerulosclerosis. A one-center study of plasma exchange effects. Transplantation. 1991;52:827.
9. Raina R, Jothi S, Vasistha P, Chakraborty R, Mangat G, et al. Post-transplant recurrence of focal segmental glomerular sclerosis: consensus statements. Kidney Int. 2024;105(3):450–63.
10. Al Shamsi, et al. Management of recurrent focal segmental glomerulosclerosis(FSGS) post renal transplantation. Transplant Rev. 2022;36(1):100675.
11. Dawson M, Ghose S, Abdelnour N, Shah R, Sreenivas A, et al. Low density lipoprotein apheresis for treatment of focal segmental Glomerulosclerosis. Hemodial Int. 2025;29(2):137–49.

12. Alasfar S, Alachkar N, et al. Rituximab and therapeutic plasma exchange in recurrent focal segmental Glomerulosclerosis post kidney transplantation. Transplantation. 2018;102(3):e115–20.
13. Karoui K, et al. Treatment of IgA nephropathy: a rapidly evolving field. J Am Soc Nephrol. 2023;35(1):103–16.
14. Trimarchi H, et al. Oxford classification of IgA nephropathy 2016: an update from the IgA nephropathy classification working group. Kidney Int. 2017;91(5):1014–21.
15. Jiang K, Pan Y, Shi L, Xu X, Bai M, Gong X, Li M. Kidney transplantation in lupus nephritis: a comprehensive review of challenges and strategies. BMC Surg. 2025;25:112.
16. Tunnicliffe D, Craig J, Tong A, Strippoli G, et al. Immunosuppressive treatment for proliferative lupus nephritis. Cochrane Database Syst Rev. 2018;2018(6):CD002922.
17. Salvadori M, Bertoni E. Complement related kidney diseases: recurrence after transplantation. World J Transplant. 2016;6(4):632–45. https://doi.org/10.5500/wjt.v6.i4.632.
18. Ahmad SB, Bomback AS. C3 Glomerulopathy: pathogenesis and treatment. Adv Chronic Kidney Dis. 2020;27(2):104–10. https://doi.org/10.1053/j.ackd.2019.12.003.
19. Ito N, Ohashi R, Nagata M. C3 glomerulopathy and current dilemmas. Clin Exp Nephrol. 2017;21(4):541–51. https://doi.org/10.1007/s10157-016-1358-5.

Post-transplant Infection-Related Kidney Injury

7

Hasan Fattah

Case 7.1

Case Summary Study

Patient: A 74-year-old female with end-stage renal disease (ESRD) secondary to Type 2 diabetes mellitus (DM2).

Transplant course: She received a deceased donor kidney transplant (DDKT) from a donor with a Kidney Donor Profile Index (KDPI) of 70%. Non-sensitized recipient, low HLA-mismatched burden 2/6.

Clinical course: The post-transplant course was complicated by BK viremia, necessitating a reduction in immunosuppression (IS). Approximately 1 year post-transplant, she developed an elevated donor-derived cell-free DNA (dd-cfDNA) level of 1.7% and de novo donor-specific antibodies (DSA) targeting multiple HLA antigens, with a total mean fluorescence intensity (MFI) of 10,000, while on reduced IS.

H. Fattah (✉)
Jacob School of Medicine and Biomedical Science,
University at Buffalo, Buffalo, NY, USA

H. Fattah, V. Cornea (eds.), *Transplantation in Practice*,
https://doi.org/10.1007/978-3-032-15908-3_7

Diagnosis

- BK virus–associated nephropathy (BKVAN) seen in the IHC (Fig. 7.1).
- Possible superimposed antibody-mediated rejection (ABMR) based on histologic and molecular findings (including g1+ and ptc2 scores) (Fig. 7.2).

Management Approach

Triggering and risk factors: The reduction in immunosuppression due to BK viremia likely triggered a rebound alloimmune response, resulting in the development of de novo DSA and elevated dd-cfDNA.

Treatment: Initiation of steroid therapy to alleviate the inflammation burden. Further reduction in immunosuppression for the management of persistent BK viremia. Mycophenolate mofetil (MMF) was discontinued. And tacrolimus was switched to cyclosporine.

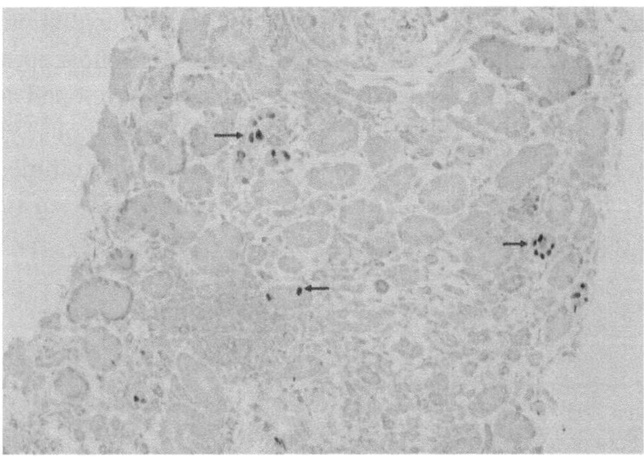

Fig. 7.1 BK-positive nuclear staining of infected tubular epithelial cells (red arrows), SV40 IHC, 20×

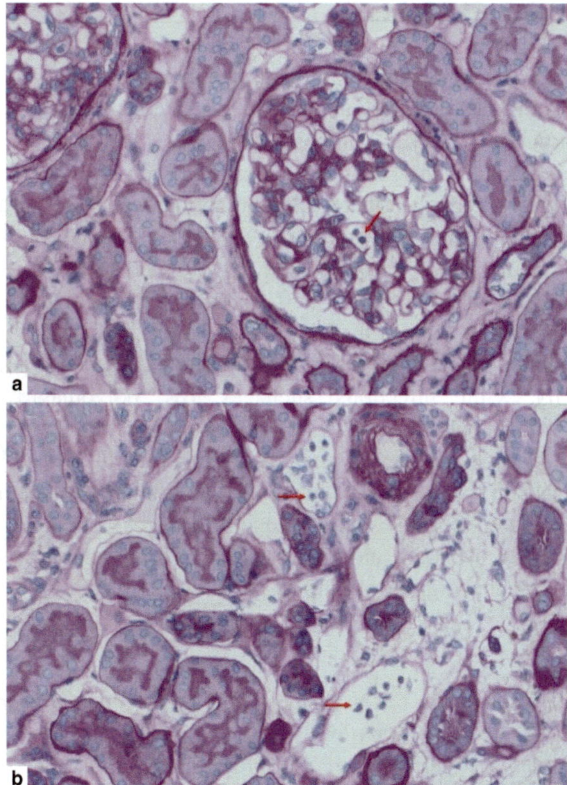

Fig. 7.2 (**a**) Glomerulitis, capillary loops with intralumenal leucocyte cell infiltrate. (red arrows). PAS, 40×. (**b**) peritubular capillaritis (red arrows), PAS, 40×

Follow-Up

- Serum creatinine remains stable throughout all the following visits at 1.3 mg/dL.
- BK virus improved but remains detectable at low grade level.
- dd-cfDNA decreased to 0.6% following steroid therapy.

Educational Insights

- In the context of polyomavirus-associated nephropathy, distinguishing between BK nephropathy and concurrent rejection (particularly ABMR) can be challenging.
- Histologic findings such as glomerulitis and peritubular capillaritis grade 1 and higher are important markers of microvascular inflammation (MVI) in kidney allograft biopsies, but these lesions are not entirely specific for antibody-mediated rejection (ABMR) [1]. The Banff classification recognizes that MVI can be seen in a variety of contexts, including T cell–mediated rejection, ischemia-reperfusion injury, and importantly, viral infections such as BK polyomavirus or cytomegalovirus, which can confound interpretation after kidney transplantation [2], and the significance of elevated dd-cfDNA in this setting remains difficult to interpret, whether it was related to viral or alloimmune injury.
- Clinical correlation and multidisciplinary judgment are essential in managing these complex cases.

Pearl 7.1

This case illustrates the challenge of balancing immunosuppression in BK virus nephropathy, where reducing therapy can trigger alloimmune activation. Careful clinical correlation is essential for diagnosis and management.

Case 7.2

Case Study Summary

Patient: A 22-year-old male with end-stage renal disease (ESRD) of unknown etiology.

Transplant: He received a living unrelated kidney transplant (LUKT); he was non-sensitized; however, this kidney was a 6/6 HLA mismatch. Induction treatment with high dose (ATG) 6 mg/

kg and steroids, followed by staying on triple immunosuppression medication, including daily prednisone 5 mg, tacrolimus with target trough levels 8–10 ng/ml, and total dose of 2 g daily mycophenolate.

Clinical Course: 5 months after transplant, the patient developed BK viremia greater than 10,000 copies/ml and a rising serum creatinine 2.5 mg/dL. Donor-specific antibodies (DSA) and donor-derived cell-free DNA (dd-cfDNA) were both undetectable.

Diagnosis

Early post-transplant AKI due to BK virus–associated nephropathy (BKVAN), viral cytopathic changes in (Fig. 7.3) and positive SV40 on ICH in (Fig. 7.4).

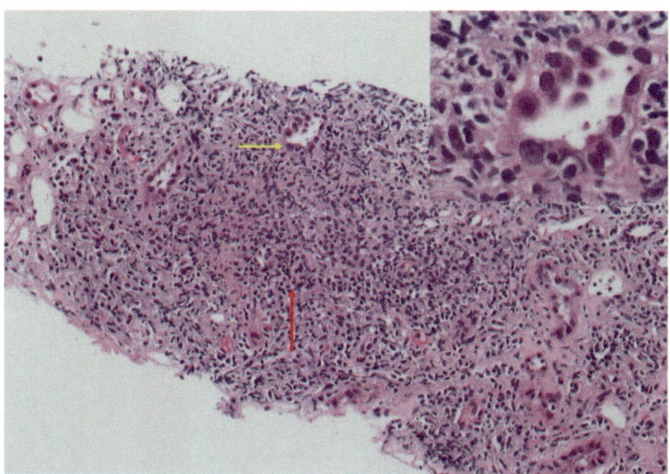

Fig. 7.3 Interstitial inflammation (red arrows), and BK viral cytopathic effect (yellow arrows) H&E, 20×. higher magnification of BK viral cytopathy in the right upper corner. H&E, 40×

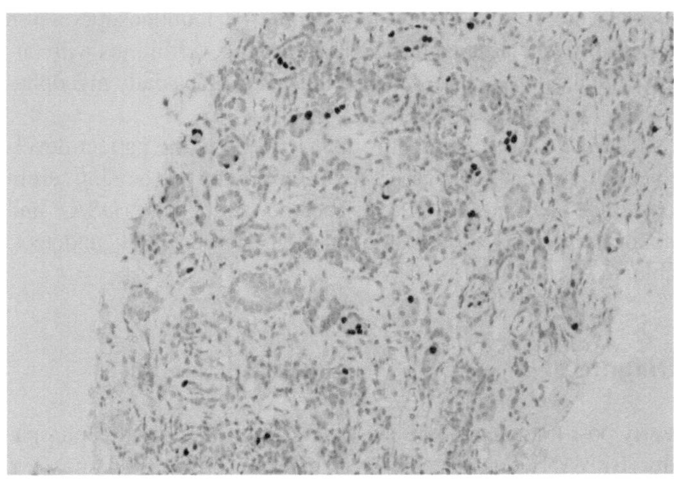

Fig. 7.4 BK-positive nuclear staining of infected tubular epithelial cells (red arrows) SV40 immunostaining, 20×

Management Approach

Risk factors many donors and recipients derived factors were identified in medical literature and were applicable to case patient; most importantly the use of steroids, high-dose lymphocyte depleting treatment, and high immunosuppressive drugs levels including tacrolimus-MMF combination in comparison to cyclosporine-MMF or m-TOR inhibitor combinations.

Treatment: Reduction in immunosuppression, both mycophenolate, and tacrolimus trough level. And weekly intravenous immunoglobulin (IVIG) at a dose of 500 mg/kg.

Follow-Up

Resolved BK viremia, persistent chronic kidney injury with a new baseline serum creatinine of 2.0 mg/dL.

Educational Insights

- BK viremia is a key surrogate marker for BKVAN, and while BK viremia can occur without nephropathy, BKVAN does not occur without viremia.
- The risk of renal allograft infection and disease correlate with the magnitude of BK viral load in blood, making post-transplant regular monitoring very critical. The following are good resources supporting this point:
  - The Kidney Disease: Improving Global Outcomes (KDIGO) guidelines state that a plasma BKV load greater than 10,000 copies/mL is associated with a high risk of BKVAN, with a reported specificity of 93% for the presence of BKVAN. The guidelines further note that kidney transplant recipients with BKV levels above this threshold are considered at risk for progression to BKVAN, even in the absence of clinical disease or elevated serum creatinine [3, 4].
  - The American Society of Transplantation also recommends that a plasma BK viremia exceeding 10,000 copies/ml reflects presumptive BKVAN and should prompt immunosuppression reduction, even without biopsy confirmation [5].

Pearl 7.2

This case emphasizes that BK viremia and BK virus–associated nephropathy (BKVAN) can occur early after transplant usually after 8–12 weeks and cause AKI. The severity of renal involvement is closely linked to the level of BK viral load in the blood.

Case 7.3

Case Study Summary

Patient: A 52-year-old female with end-stage renal disease (ESRD) secondary to diabetes mellitus.

Transplant course: She received a deceased donor kidney transplant (DDKT), calculated panel reactive antibody (cPRA) 28%, 0/6 HLA mismatch. Induction treatment with ATG 4 mg/kg, steroids and followed by tacrolimus-MMF combination treatment.

Clinical Course: Two months after transplant, the patient developed severe BK viremia and persistently elevated serum creatinine of 2.0 mg/dL. Donor-derived cell-free DNA (dd-cfDNA) and de novo donor-specific antibodies (DSA) were undetectable.

Diagnosis

- Polyomavirus-associated nephropathy (BKVAN) based on LM and IHC (Fig. 7.5).
- Suspicious changes on biopsy for ABMR (Fig. 7.6), molecular diagnostics (MMDx) confirmed mild antibody-mediated rejection (ABMR) and severe T cell–mediated rejection (TCMR).

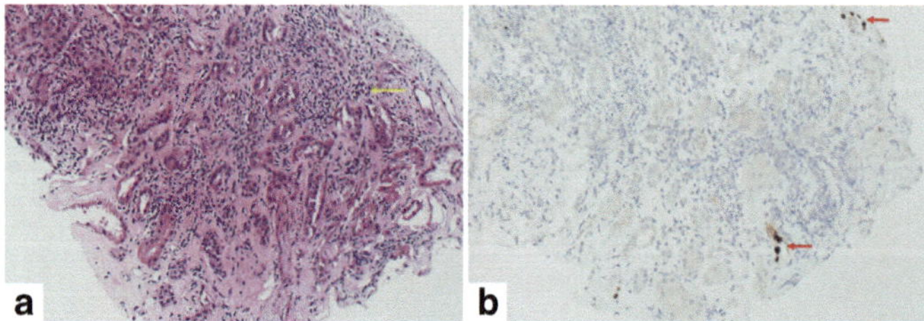

Fig. 7.5 (**a**) Interstitial inflammation, mild tubulitis, with no evidence of cytopathic effect (yellow arrow) H&E, 20×. (**b**) BK positive nuclear staining (red arrows), SV40 IHC, 20×

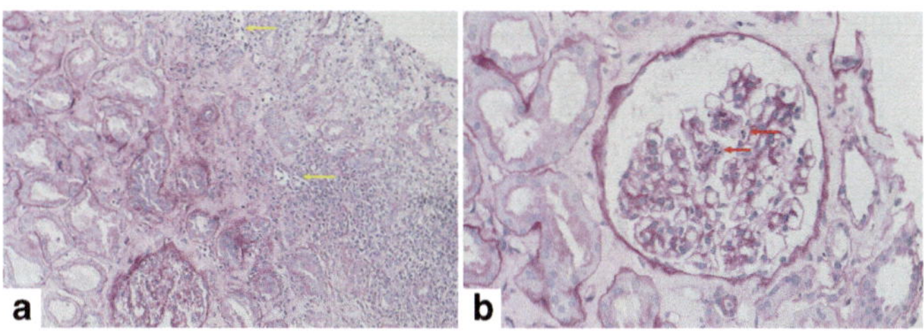

Fig. 7.6 (**a**) peritubular capillirits PTC 1 (yellow arrows) PAS, 20×. (**b**) glomerulitis g1, PAS, 20×

Management Approach

Triggering Factors

- Insufficient cellular immune control due to high immunosuppression level is a key contributor to BKVAN pathogenesis.
- Additional risk factors may include high-risk serostatus and donor BKPyV viruria prior to transplantation.

Treatment: Reduction of immunosuppression, weekly IVIG of the dose 500 mg/kg for total 4 weeks, with weak response to the above treatment, and after ruling out active rejection, she received BK-specific viral therapy using immune T-cell therapy (VST) [6].

Follow-Up

- Graft function stable to slightly improved. Serum creatinine decreased to 1.8 mg/dL.
- BK viremia resolved.

Educational Insights

- Transcriptomic analysis and BK nephropathy: Multiple studies using microarray and RNA-sequencing approaches have shown that BKVAN and acute rejection (both T cell–mediated and antibody-mediated) share upregulation of immune response genes, including those related to cytotoxic T cells, interferon signaling, chemokines, and macrophage activation [7, 8].

- Histologic markers of concurrent TCMR and BK nephropathy are not uncommon; distinguishing between them is challenging and requires expert histopathologic evaluation.
- One diagnostic approach suggests that areas of inflammation with negative SV40 staining may indicate concurrent acute rejection, rather than viral injury alone.

Pearl 7.3

BKVAN and acute rejection share similar immune gene expression profiles, making them difficult to distinguish. Inflammation without SV40 staining may suggest rejection, underscoring the need for expert pathology review.

Case 7.4

Case Study Summary

Patient: A 53-year-old male with end stage renal disease (ESRD) secondary to granulomatosis with polyangiitis (GPA).

Transplant course: He received a donation after circulatory death (DCD) kidney transplant with a KDPI of 73% and a 4/6 HLA mismatch. He received induction with ATG and steroids, followed by tacrolimus-MMF combination. Immunologic risk: cPRA 0%.

Clinical Course: prolonged delayed graft function (DGF), prompting a kidney biopsy about 4 weeks post-transplant.

Diagnosis

Kidney biopsy confirmed adenovirus nephritis. Nonspecific viral cytopathic in (Fig. 7.7) and positive adenovirus by IHC (Fig. 7.8).

Management Approach

Triggering Factors

- High immunosuppressive burden.
- Potential high donor to recipient adenovirus risk status.

Treatment: Reduction in immunosuppression, weekly Intravenous immunoglobulin (IVIG) dose of 500 mg/kg, and Cidofovir antiviral therapy.

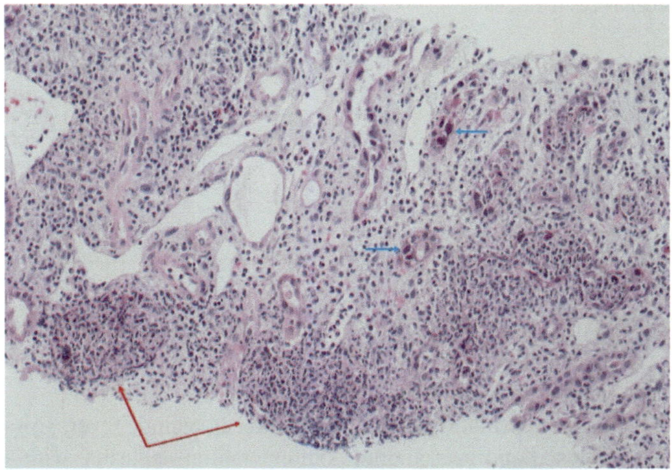

Fig. 7.7 Nuclear viral cytopathic effect (blue arrows), ATN, hemorrhage and increased PMNs in the interstitial infiltrate (red arrows) H&E, 20×

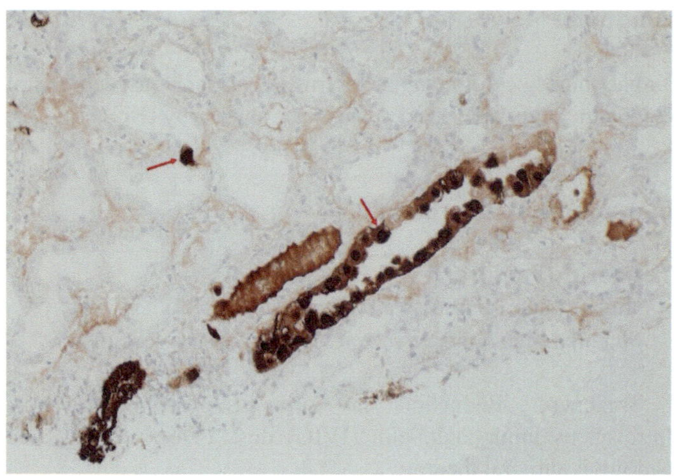

Fig. 7.8 Adenovirus nuclear staining of infected epithelial cells (red arrows). Adenovirus IHC, 20×

Follow-Up

The patient unfortunately developed primary graft non-function and returned to dialysis.

Educational Insights

- Post-transplant adenovirus infection presents variably in the first 3 months after transplantation and may be due to primary infection or reactivation.
- Clinical presentation is diverse [9] and can include fever, gross hematuria, and necrotizing tubulointerstitial nephritis, with a cellular infiltrate predominantly of neutrophils and macrophages—features that can mimic bacterial infection. However, sometimes it can present with persistent delayed graft function like in this unique case.

- Histologically, adenovirus may resemble BK virus with viral inclusion bodies, but is distinguished by foci of granulomatous inflammation, prominent tubular necrosis, and interstitial hemorrhage [10].
- Reduction in immunosuppression is the cornerstone of treatment; antiviral therapy is reserved for disseminated or refractory cases.

Pearl 7.4

Adenovirus nephritis is rare; it can mimic BK virus but often presents with necrosis, hemorrhage, and neutrophil-rich infiltrates. Early diagnosis and reduction in immunosuppression are critical to prevent graft loss.

Case 7.5

Case Study Summary

*Patient***:** A 70-year-old male with end-stage renal disease (ESRD) of unknown etiology in the setting of long-standing history of hypertension.

*Transplant course***:** He received a deceased donor kidney transplant (DDKT) from a donor with KDPI of 50%; he was slightly sensitized with panel reactive antibody (cPRA) of 25% and received ATG and steroids induction followed by prednisone and Tac-MMF combination therapy.

Clinical course: Five months post-transplant, the patient developed acute kidney injury (AKI) with a urine protein-to-creatinine ratio (UPC) of 1 g/g and BK viral load of 2.7 million copies/mL, later peaking at 5 million. No donor-specific antibodies (DSA) were detected. Kidney biopsy revealed BK virus–associated nephropathy (BKVAN) class II. Donor-derived cell-free DNA (dd-cfDNA) peaked at 0.8% during the height of viremia (Fig. 7.9).

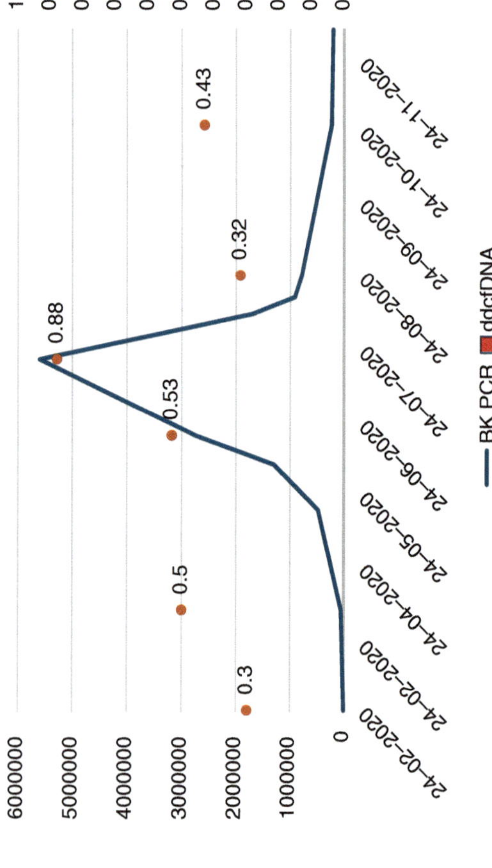

Fig. 7.9 dd-cfDNA titer and BK copies peak and resolution levels timeline

Diagnosis

BKVAN, class II, both nonspecific viral cytopathic changes (Fig. 7.10), and positive SV 40 on IHC (Fig. 7.11).

Management Approach

Triggering factors: Multifactorial, high immunosuppressive burden, older age, and male sex—all associated with increased risk of BKVAN.

Treatment: Reduction in immunosuppression, weekly intravenous immunoglobulin (IVIG), conversion from tacrolimus to cyclosporine.

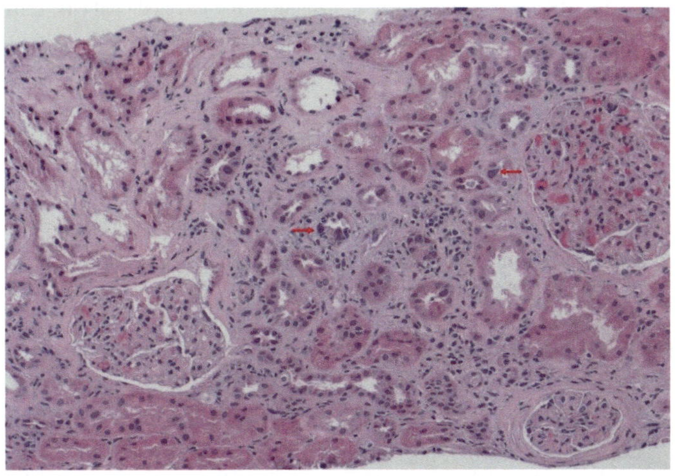

Fig. 7.10 BK nuclear cytopathic effect, (red arrows) H&E, 20×

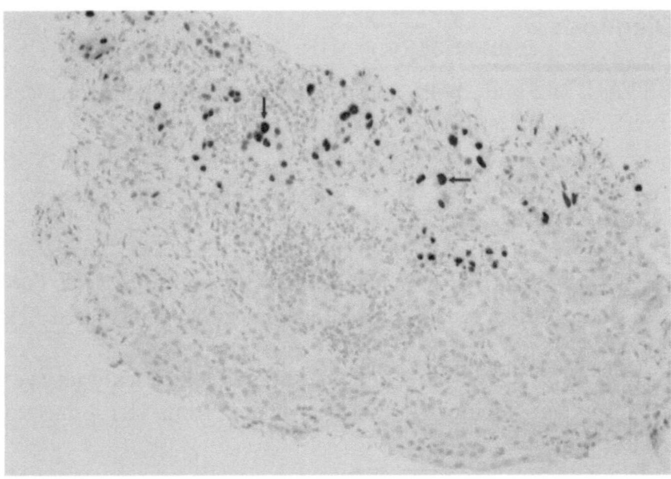

Fig. 7.11 BK virus positive nuclear staining of the infected epithelial cells (red arrows) SV-40 IHC, 20×

Follow-Up

- dd-cfDNA decreased with resolution of BK viremia (Fig. 7.9).
- Patient now has stable CKD stage 4, maintaining consistent graft function 5 years post-transplant.

Educational Insights

- Donor-derived cell-free DNA (dd-cfDNA) is a promising biomarker for identifying and monitoring BK virus–associated nephropathy (BKVAN). However, its clinical utility may be nuanced by the overlap in allograft injury pathways between BKVAN and acute rejection [11].

- It may assist in evaluating injury severity, tracking response to therapy, and refining the clinical interpretation of BK PCR titers.
- Plasma dd-cfDNA rises in BKVAN, but the magnitude of increase is generally less than that seen in antibody-mediated rejection and is not reliably different from TCMR.

Pearl 7.5

This case highlights the utility of donor-derived cell-free DNA (dd-cfDNA) in monitoring BK virus–associated nephropathy (BKVAN). dd-cfDNA levels correlated with BK viral load and injury severity, supporting its role as a complementary tool to BK PCR for diagnosis and response to treatment.

Case 7.6

Case Study Summary

Patient: A 73-year-old female with ESRD of unknown etiology.

Transplant course: She received a deceased donor kidney transplant (DDKT) from a donor with kidney donor profile index (KDPI) of 74%; recipient's cPRA was 17%. She received ATG and steroids induction followed by daily prednisone and Tac-MMF combination treatment. Immediate graft function was achieved with a nadir serum creatinine of 1.5 mg/dL.

Clinical Course: Two months post-transplant, the patient developed severe acute kidney injury (AKI) requiring hemodialysis. Imaging revealed a perinephric fluid collection concerning for lymphocele, which was drained. Despite intervention, renal function did not recover, prompting a biopsy. Serologic workup was negative, but urinalysis showed pyuria, and culture grew normal skin flora.

Diagnosis

Acute pyelonephritis of the transplanted kidney based on biopsy analysis, prominent interstitial infiltrates of PMNs seen (Figs. 7.12 and 7.13).

Management Approach

Risk factors: Potential contributors include typical urinary tract infection (UTI) risk factors, with prior interventional drainage possibly predisposing to infection.

Treatment started an antibiotic course.

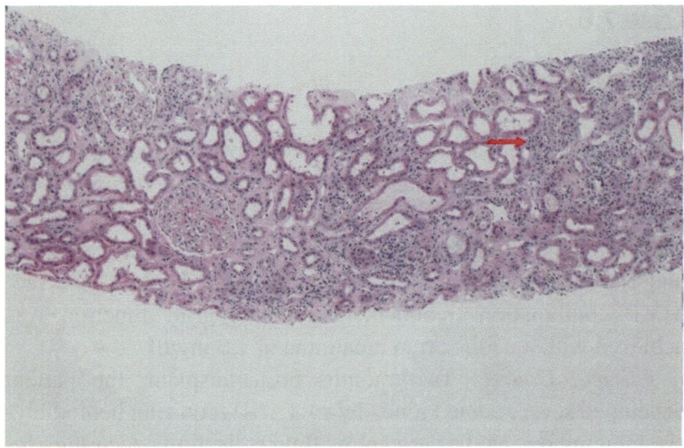

Fig. 7.12 Interstitial mixed inflammatory infiltrate with PMNs (polymorphonuclear neutrophils), red arrow. H&E, 10×

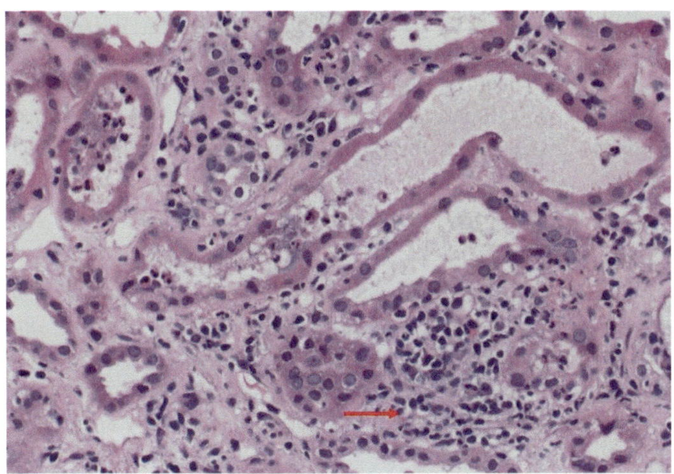

Fig. 7.13 Higher magnification, interstitial mixed inflammatory infiltrate with PMNs (red arrow). H&E, 40×

Follow-Up

- Renal function improved with antibiotics and lymphocele resolution.
- At 5 years post-transplant, kidney function remains stable with serum creatinine of 1.0 mg/dL and GFR of 60 mL/min.

Educational Insights

- Acute transplant pyelonephritis can present subtly due to immunosuppression, often without classic symptoms such as fever or dysuria.
- Risk factors include female sex, diabetes, high immunosuppression levels, urinary tract abnormalities such as ureter strictures, or prolonged indwelling instrumentations [12].
- AKI may be the only presenting feature, particularly in the early post-transplant period.

- Pathologically acute pyelonephritis is characterized by neutrophils tubulitis, neutrophils casts and predominantly polymorphonuclear neutrophils (PMNs) interstitial infiltrates, unlike the distinct lymphocyte-predominant infiltrate of acute rejection and the viral cytopathic changes seen in viral nephropathies.

Pearl 7.6

This case highlights that acute transplant pyelonephritis can present atypically, often without fever or urinary symptoms, and may initially manifest as isolated AKI. Distinguishing it from acute rejection could be challenging and requires careful clinical, microbiologic, and histologic correlation, especially early post-transplant.

Case 7.7

Case Study Summary

Patient: A 59-year-old male with ESRD secondary to Type 2 diabetes mellitus.

Transplant course: He received a living unrelated kidney transplant (LUKT) with a 5/6 HLA mismatch and 0% panel reactive antibodies (cPRA). CMV status donor positive to recipient negative. Induction treatment with ATG (total 4.5 mg/kg), and steroids followed by maintenance therapy with tacrolimus (target trough 4–6 ng/mL), MMF, and prednisone 5 mg daily.

Clinical course: Seven months post-transplant, the patient developed BK viremia, peaking at 160,000 copies/mL; he had persistent viremia despite appropriate reduction in immunosuppression. Kidney function remained at baseline (serum creatinine 1.5 mg/dL), and urinalysis was clean.

Diagnosis

A kidney biopsy confirmed BK virus–associated nephropathy (BKVAN), class II (Figs. 7.14 and 7.15).

Management Approach

Risk factors: Likely multifactorial, including immunosuppression intensity, CMV high-risk status, and HLA mismatch.

Treatment: Initial reduction in immunosuppression, and due to unsatisfactory response to this treatment, patient was opted to received virus-specific T-cell (VST) therapy.

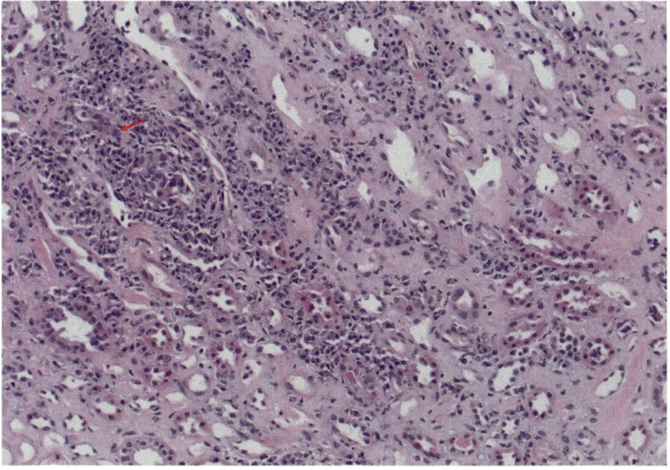

Fig. 7.14 BK viral nuclear cytopathic effect in the infected tubular epithelial cells, (red arrow). H&E, 20×

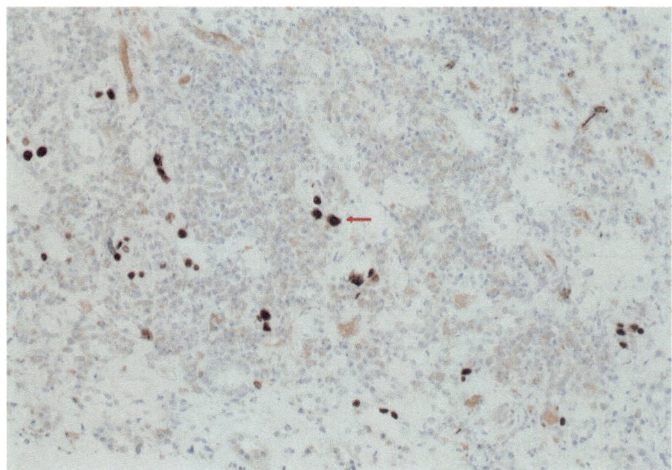

Fig. 7.15 BK virus immunostaining positive nuclear the infected tubular epithelial cells, (red arrow), SV40, 20×

Follow-Up

- One-year post-transplant, BK viral load declined to 39,000 copies/mL and continued to decline over time,
- Patient continues VST therapy with stable renal function.

Educational Insights

- Reduction in immunosuppression remains the first-line treatment for BK viremia and BKVAN.
- Virus-specific T-cell therapy (VSTs) may be particularly valuable when immunosuppression reduction is inadequate or contraindicated due to high rejection risk.
- Virus-specific T-cell therapy (VST) has shown promise as a safe and potentially effective option for controlling BK viremia in kidney transplant recipients, especially in cases refrac-

tory to immunosuppression reduction, with response rates of 45–86% in some studies and minimal reported toxicity or allograft rejection [13, 14].

Pearl 7.7

In high-risk transplant patients, BK nephropathy may not respond to immunosuppression reduction alone; virus-specific T-cell therapy offers a valuable alternative to control viremia without increasing rejection risk.

Case 7.8

Case Study Summary

Patient: A 64-year-old male with end-stage renal disease (ESRD) due to focal segmental glomerulosclerosis (FSGS).

Transplant course: He received a living unrelated kidney transplant (LUKT), later complicated by BK virus–associated nephropathy (BKVAN).

Initial Management: Treated with IVIG and reduction in immunosuppression. Despite minimal immunosuppression, BK viremia improved but never fully resolved. Baseline creatinine stabilized at 2.0 mg/dL.

Subsequent events: The patient developed microscopic hematuria, prompting a urologic evaluation. Cystoscopy and biopsy revealed in situ high-grade papillary urothelial carcinoma located in the left and anterior bladder wall. Notably, tumor cells stained positive for SV40, indicating a potential polyomavirus (PyV)–associated malignancy.

Diagnosis

BK virus–associated high-grade urothelial carcinoma (Figs. 7.16 and 7.17).

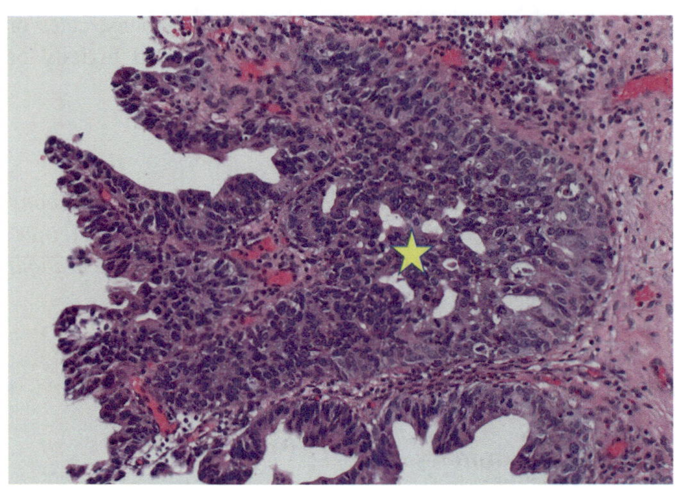

Fig. 7.16 High grade urothelial carcinoma (yellow star), H&E, 20×

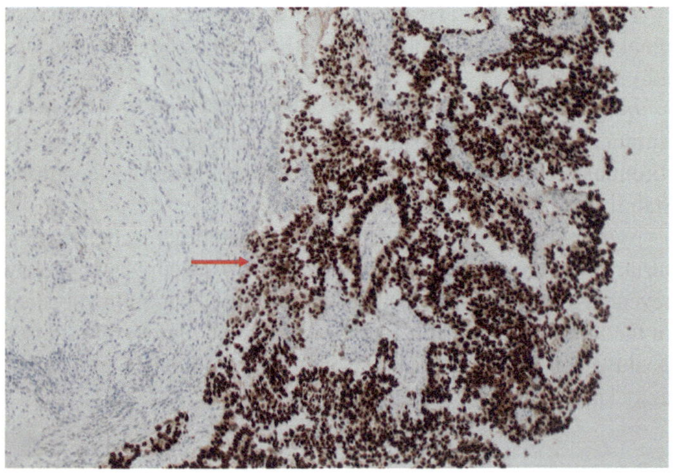

Fig. 7.17 Immunostain for BK virus, positive nuclear staining in the neoplastic cells (red arrow), SV-40, 10×

Management Approach

Risk factors: Immunosuppression, BK polyomavirus, with chronic infection and viral oncogene expression contributing to malignant transformation.

Treatment: Intravesical chemotherapy with cisplatin and gemcitabine.

Follow-Up

At 8 years post-transplant, the patient has stable graft function, with well-controlled BK viremia and no recurrence of cancer.

Educational Insights

- Polyomaviruses, including BK virus, can rarely contribute to urothelial carcinoma through chronic infection and direct oncogenic mechanisms, including the expression of viral oncoproteins and promotion of genomic instability [15].
- There is accumulating evidence that polyomaviruses, particularly BK virus, contribute to significantly increased incidence of urinary tract cancers, including bladder and upper tract urothelial carcinomas, compared to those without BKPyVAN [16].
- In the absence of immune clearance, persistently infected epithelial cells may undergo malignant transformation, resulting in SV40-positive PyV-associated tumors.

Pearl 7.8

This case illustrates that chronic BK virus infection, though typically associated with nephropathy, can rarely lead to urothelial carcinoma through viral oncogenesis. Persistent infection and lack of immune clearance may allow BK virus to induce malignant transformation, highlighting the importance of monitoring unexplained hematuria in transplant recipients with ongoing BK viremia.

Case 7.9

Special thanks to Dr. John Tomaszewski for kindly providing case images that helped bring this subject to life.

Case Study Summary

Patient: A 62-year-old female with end-stage renal disease (ESRD) in the setting of hypertensive and diabetic nephrosclerosis underwent a preemptive deceased donor kidney transplant (DDKT).

Transplant course: Her calculated PRA was 0%. Induction immunosuppression consisted of thymoglobulin (ATG) and corticosteroids. She was noted to have delayed graft function and was discharged on dialysis and wound infection requiring treatment with IV antibiotics.

Clinical course: Two weeks post-transplant, the patient was admitted with weakness, positive blood cultures for *Candida glabrata* and was treated with micafungin, resulting in initial clinical improvement. However, she continued to experience DGF prompting a renal allograft biopsy at 4 weeks post-transplant.

Diagnosis

- Urine cultures were negative for fungal organisms, or pyuria, making lower urinary tract infection less likely.
- Transplant fungal nephritis, this diagnosis was established based on:
  - Prior positive blood cultures for *Candida glabrata.*
  - Histopathological findings from the kidney biopsy, which demonstrated:
    - Multifocal mixed lymphocytic and neutrophilic interstitial inflammation (Fig. 7.18).
    - Focally vigorous neutrophilic tubulitis involving 25% of the sampled cortex and the medulla.

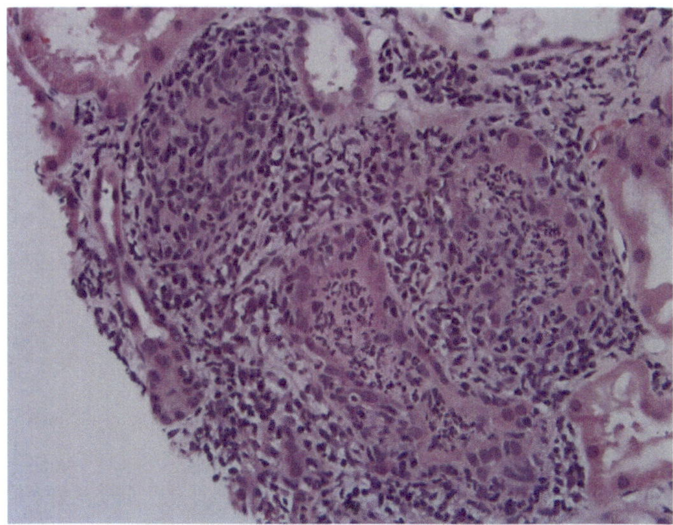

Fig. 7.18 Mixed lymphocytic and neutrophilic interstitial inflammation and tubulitis (microabscesses), H&E 40×

- Tubular yeast forms on Periodic Acid-Schiff (PAS) staining, consistent with active fungal nephritis (Figs. 7.19 and 7.20).

Management Approach

Risk factors contributing to fungal infection in this patient are numerous included: diabetes mellitus, use of antibiotics, and lymphocyte-depleting induction therapy (ATG) [17].

Therapeutic adjustments included:

- Transition to high-dose oral fluconazole, guided by *C. glabrata* susceptibility.
- Reduction of immunosuppression**:**
  - Mycophenolate mofetil (MMF) was held, and tacrolimus target level was reduced.

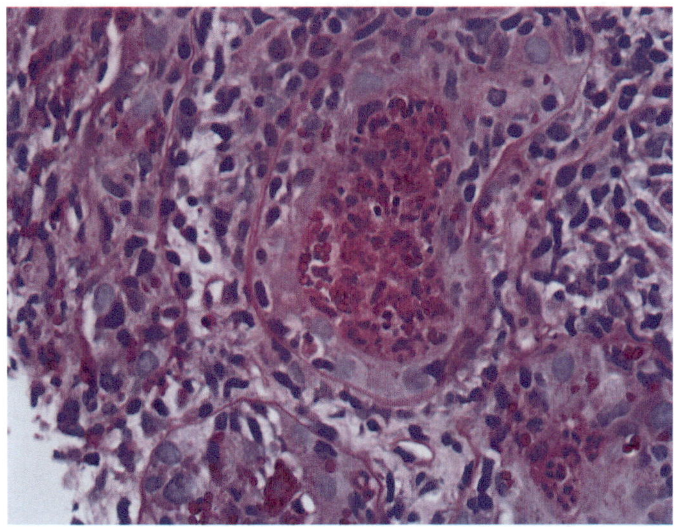

Fig. 7.19 Tubular yeast forms on Periodic Acid-Schiff (PAS) staining, consistent with active fungal nephritis, PAS, 40×

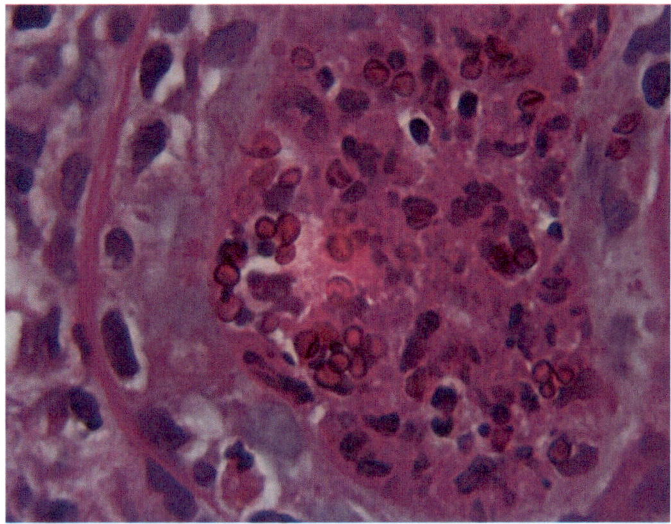

Fig. 7.20 Higher power demonstration of the tubular yeast forms on Periodic Acid-Schiff (PAS)

Follow-Up

At the time of follow-up:

- The patient had been weaned off hemodialysis and creatinine on most recent visits was 1.5.
- Continued to receive oral fluconazole.
- A repeat renal biopsy performed 4 weeks after changing to fluconazole revealed minimal inflammation and a complete resolution of fungal nephritis.

Educational Insights

- Fungal nephritis following kidney transplantation is rare but clinically significant. The overall prevalence of invasive fungal infections (IFIs) in kidney transplant recipients ranges from 2–10%, with *Candida* and *Aspergillus* species being the most common pathogens [18].
- Renal parenchymal involvement (i.e., true fungal nephritis) is less common than lower urinary tract fungal infections, though both may coexist.
- For *Candida* nephritis, fluconazole is typically the first-line therapy if the organism is susceptible, due to its excellent urinary penetration [19].
- For fluconazole-resistant *Candida* species (e.g., *Candida krusei*), alternative agents include liposomal amphotericin B or flucytosine, though both have significant nephrotoxic potential, especially in transplant recipients.
- Echinocandins such as micafungin are generally avoided in urinary tract infections due to poor urinary excretion but may be considered in specific cases based on systemic needs and individual susceptibility profiles.
- Mortality rates for IFIs in transplant recipients remain high, ranging from 15–71% depending on the pathogen and timing of diagnosis.
- Prompt recognition, early antifungal therapy, and modification of immunosuppression are key to improving clinical outcomes.

References

1. Sablik M. Microvascular inflammation of kidney allografts and clinical outcomes. N Engl J Med. 2024; https://doi.org/10.1056/NEJMoa2408835.
2. Metter C. Pathology of the kidney allograft. Semin Diagn Pathol. 2020;37(3):148–53. https://doi.org/10.1053/j.semdp.2020.03.005.
3. KDIGO. KDIGO clinical practice guideline for the care of kidney transplant recipients. Am J Transplant. 2009;9(Suppl 3):S1–155. https://doi.org/10.1111/j.1600-6143.2009.02834.
4. Kasiske BL, et al. KDIGO clinical practice guideline for the care of kidney transplant recipients: a summary. Kidney Int. 2010;77(4):299–311.
5. Hirsch HH. BK polyomavirus in solid organ transplantation-guidelines from the American society of transplantation infectious diseases community of practice. Clin Transpl. 2019;33(9):e13528. https://doi.org/10.1111/ctr.13528.
6. Nelson A. Virus-specific T-cell therapy to treat BK polyomavirus infection in bone marrow and solid organ transplant recipients. Blood Adv. 2020;4(22):5745–54.
7. Lubetzky M. Genomics of BK viremia in kidney transplant recipients. Transplantation. 2014;97(4):451–6. https://doi.org/10.1097/01.TP.0000437432.35227.3e.
8. Sigdel TK. Intragraft antiviral-specific gene expression as a distinctive transcriptional signature for studies in polyomavirus-associated nephropathy. Transplantation. 2016;100(10):2062–70. https://doi.org/10.1097/TP.0000000000001214.
9. Swathi Kiran P. Adenovirus nephritis in adult kidney allograft recipients: a systematic review of literature. Infection. 2025;53(1):25–37. https://doi.org/10.1007/s15010-024-02455-y.
10. Jagannathan G. The pathologic spectrum of adenovirus nephritis in the kidney allograft. Kidney Int. 2023;103(2):378–90. https://doi.org/10.1016/j.kint.2022.10.025.
11. Wen J. Detection of BK polyomavirus-associated nephropathy using plasma graft-derived cell-free DNA: development of a novel algorithm from programmed monitoring. Front Immunol. 2022;13:1006970. https://doi.org/10.3389/fimmu.2022.1006970.
12. Fiorentino M. Updates on urinary tract infections in kidney transplantation. J Nephrol. 2019;32(5):751–61. https://doi.org/10.1007/s40620-019-00585-3.
13. Anand M. Viral specific T cell therapy in kidney transplant recipients - a single-center experience. Transpl Infect Dis. 2023;25(6):e14179. https://doi.org/10.1111/tid.14179.
14. Alkan B. Advances in virus-specific T-cell therapy for polyomavirus infections: a comprehensive review. Int J Antimicrob Agents. 2024;64(5):107333. https://doi.org/10.1016/j.ijantimicag.2024.107333.

15. Gupta G. Treatment for presumed BK polyomavirus nephropathy and risk of urinary tract cancers among kidney transplant recipients in the United States. Am J Transplant. 2018;18(1):245–52. https://doi.org/10.1111/ajt.14530.
16. Li YJ. High incidence and early onset of urinary tract cancers in patients with BK polyomavirus associated nephropathy. Viruses. 2021;13(3):476. https://doi.org/10.3390/v13030476.
17. Seok H. Invasive fungal diseases in kidney transplant recipients: risk factors for mortality. J Clin Med. 2020;9(6):E1824. https://doi.org/10.3390/jcm9061824.
18. Mazzitelli M. Fungal infections in kidney transplant recipients: a comprehensive narrative review. Microorganisms. 2025;13(1):207. https://doi.org/10.3390/microorganisms13010207.
19. Paya CV. Fungal infections in solid organ transplantation. Clin Infect Dis. 1993;16(5):677–88. https://doi.org/10.1093/clind/16.5.677.

Post-transplant Metabolic-Related Kidney Injury

8

Hasan Fattah

Case 8.1

Case Study Summary

Patient: is a 70-year-old male with end stage renal disease (ESRD) due to obstructive nephropathy and comorbid short bowel syndrome.

Transplant course: he received a deceased donor kidney transplant (DDKT) from a donor with kidney donor profile index (KDPI) of 22%, he was highly sensitized with cPRA 91%, and the donor/recipient HLA mismatch was 4/6. Induction treatment included ATG 6 mg/kg, steroids, and maintenance treatment with Tac-MMF combination.

Clinical course: post-transplant, the patient developed persistent acute kidney injury (AKI) with a serum creatinine of 3.0 mg/dL, prompting two biopsies on postoperative days 25 and 55. Laboratory findings included mild hypercalcemia, elevated PTH at 338 pg/mL, and urine pH >8. DEXA scan revealed osteoporosis, and a Tc-99m sestamibi scan showed subtle focal uptake suggestive of a possible parathyroid adenoma.

H. Fattah (✉)
Jacob School of Medicine and Biomedical Science,
University at Buffalo, Buffalo, NY, USA

H. Fattah, V. Cornea (eds.), *Transplantation in Practice*,
https://doi.org/10.1007/978-3-032-15908-3_8

Diagnosis

- Persistent acute tubular necrosis (ATN) (Fig. 8.1).
- Calcium phosphate crystal deposition likely secondary to ATN (Fig. 8.2).
- No evidence of rejection.

Management Approach

Triggering factors: Short bowel syndrome leading to electrolyte imbalances and volume depletion, also hyperparathyroidism contributing to hypercalcemia and calcium phosphate deposition.

Treatment: Daily intravenous fluid administration for volume expansion, cinacalcet for possible tertiary hyperparathyroidism.

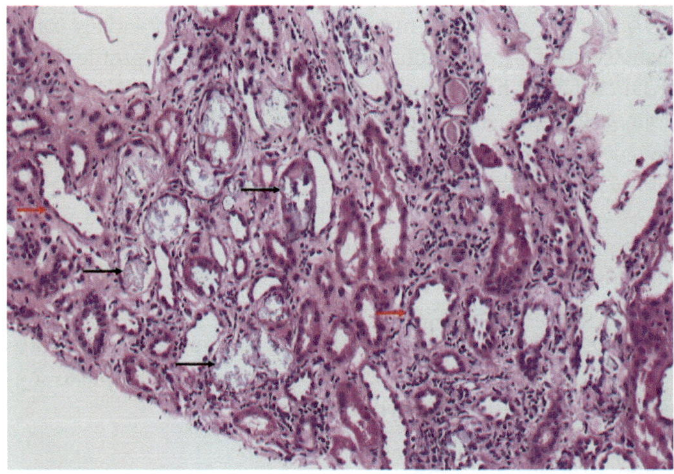

Fig. 8.1 ATN evidenced by epithelial cell simplification (red arrows), and intracellular calcium phosphate crystal deposition (black arrows), H&E, 20×

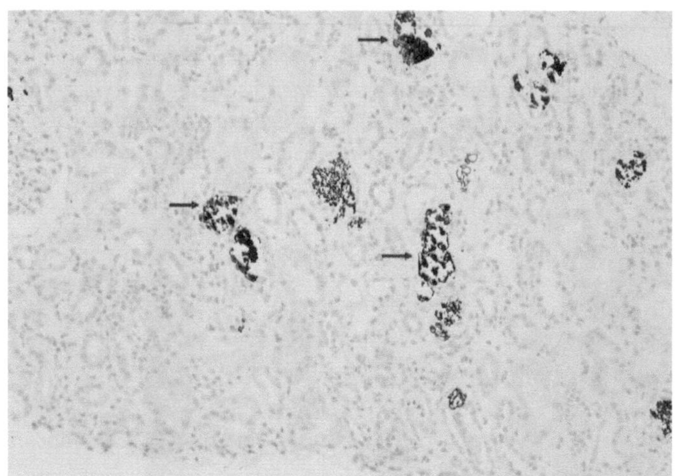

Fig. 8.2 Calcium phosphate crystals (red arrows) Von Kossa, 20×

Follow-Up

At 1-year post-transplant, the patient has stable graft function with a creatinine of 1.5 mg/dL.

Educational Insights

- Kidney transplantation in recipients with short bowel syndrome (SBS) is associated with acceptable short and midterm outcomes [1].
- Calcium phosphate deposition due to elevated urine PH in the setting of overt or incomplete distal renal tubular acidosis is a possible contributor to graft injury.
- Volume expansion with IV fluids is a key intervention to prevent or mitigate crystal-induced injury.
- Careful metabolic evaluation is essential to distinguish non-rejection causes of AKI.

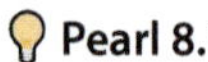

Kidney transplant is not absolutely contraindicated in recipients with history of short bowel syndrome, metabolic complications, and ATN due to volume depletion can lead to graft injury. Volume expansion with home IV fluids is essential to prevent such damage; thorough metabolic evaluation is critical to diagnose these non-rejection causes of AKI.

Case 8.2

Case Study Summary

Patient: A 55-year-old with ESRD secondary to Type 1 diabetes mellitus.

Transplant course: He received a deceased donor kidney transplant (DDKT) from a donor with KDPI of 76%, he was not sensitized his cPRA0%, and he received ATG and steroids for induction followed by daily prednisone and Tac-MMF combination immunosuppression.

Clinical Course: The patient experienced delayed graft function (DGF) post-transplant with a negative workup for rejection and a normal initial renal ultrasound. A biopsy at 4 weeks post-transplant revealed acute tubular necrosis (ATN) with prominent polarized calcium oxalate (CaOx) crystal deposition. Serum oxalate level was within normal range.Repeat renal ultrasound with Doppler and angiography identified significant torsion-related iliac artery stenosis, leading to transplant renal artery stenosis (TRAS). The patient underwent iliac artery stenting, leading to rapid improvement in renal function and resolution of DGF.

Diagnosis

- Transplant renal artery stenosis (TRAS).
- Acute tubular necrosis (ATN) with secondary calcium oxalate deposition (Fig. 8.3) and birefringent intratubular calcium oxalate crystal as seen under polarized light in (Fig. 8.4).

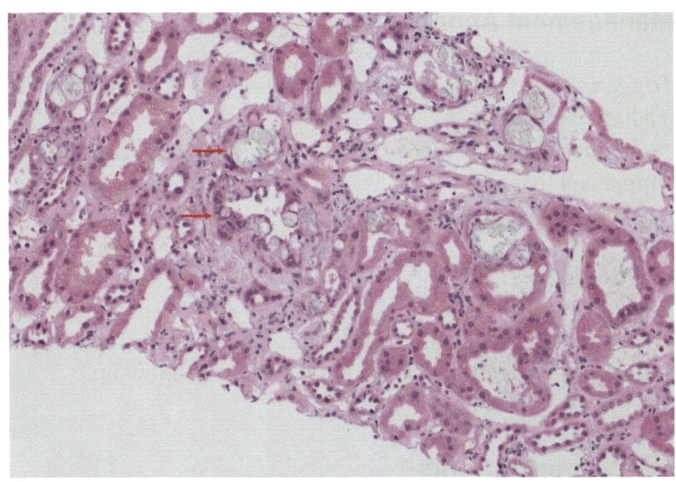

Fig. 8.3 Intratubular fan-shape calcium oxalate crystals (red arrows) H&E, 20×

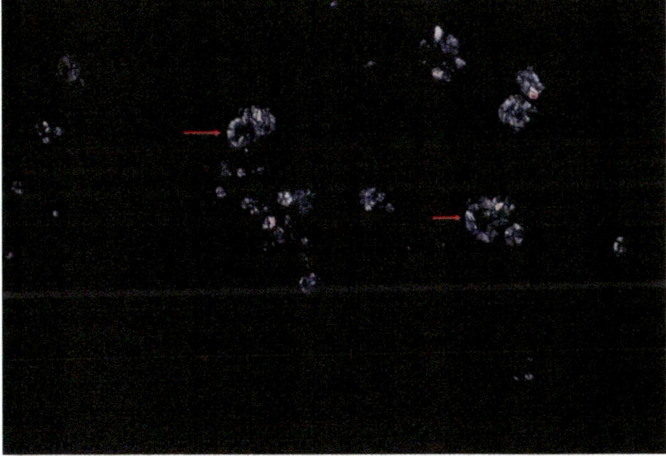

Fig. 8.4 The same intratubular calcium oxalate crystal, now birefringent under polarized light 20×

Management Approach

Triggering factor: Surgical technique–related vascular torsion leading to underperfusion.

Treatment: Endovascular iliac artery stent placement, dual antiplatelet therapy.

Follow-Up

The patient has maintained stable graft function with a serum creatinine of 1.3 mg/dL at 3 years post-transplant follow-up.

Educational Insights

- In transplant recipients, secondary CaOx deposition may result from transient hyperoxaluria, often triggered by sudden improvements in GFR after prolonged ESRD and systemic oxalate accumulation [2].
- CaOx deposition in renal transplant biopsy is a frequent finding and may be secondary to any of the causes seen in native kidney; however, it is often a consequence of ATN [3].
- Volume under perfusion and ischemic injury can exacerbate CaOx deposition and ATN.
- TRAS can present subtly with DGF and should be suspected when renal function fails to improve and acute alloimmune injury is ruled out; imaging with duplex ultrasound and angiography is key.
- Timely vascular intervention can reverse ischemia-related injury and restore graft function.

 **Pearl 8.2**

In kidney transplant recipients, delayed graft function with calcium oxalate deposition may reflect transient hyperoxaluria secondary to improved GFR after ESRD. This deposition is often a consequence—not a cause—of tubular injury,

References

1. Abou Diwan E. Short bowel syndrome and kidney transplantation: challenges, outcomes, and the use of Teduglutide. Case Rep Transplant. 2020;2020:8819345. https://doi.org/10.1155/2020/8819345.
2. Truong LD. Calcium oxalate deposition in renal allografts: morphologic spectrum and clinical implications. Am J Transplant. 2004;4(8):1338–44. https://doi.org/10.1111/j.1600-6143.2004.00511.x.
3. Geraghty R. Calcium oxalate crystal deposition in the kidney: identification, causes and consequences. Urolithiasis. 2020;48(5):377–84. https://doi.org/10.1007/s00240-020-01202-w.

9 Post-transplant TMA/ aHUS-Related Kidney Injury

Hasan Fattah

Case 9.1

Case Study Summary

Patient: A 42-year-old male with CKD stage 5 due to IgA nephropathy.

Transplant course: He underwent preemptive living unrelated kidney transplant (LUKT) from a donor with 5/6 HLA mismatch. He was sensitized (cPRA 73%) at the time of transplant. Induction treatment included ATG and steroids; maintenance was a daily prednisone and combo of Tac-MMF at maximal doses due to high immunologic risk.

Post-transplant course: The patient developed slow graft function and laboratory evidence of microangiopathic hemolytic anemia (MAHA), including schistocytes on peripheral smear and a mildly decreased complement level C4 to 10 mg/dL.

Other laboratory results:

- Direct antiglobulin test (DAT): Negative.
- HIT antibody: Undetectable.
- ADAMTS13 activity: Normal.

H. Fattah (✉)
Jacob School of Medicine and Biomedical Science,
University at Buffalo, Buffalo, NY, USA

H. Fattah, V. Cornea (eds.), *Transplantation in Practice*,
https://doi.org/10.1007/978-3-032-15908-3_9

- Atypical HUS genetic panel: Negative except for a Variant of Uncertain Significance (VUS) in exon 8 of MCP/CD46.
- DSA and viral/infectious serologies: Undetectable.
- A biopsy performed on day 7 post-transplant revealed thrombotic microangiopathy (TMA) and severe acute tubular necrosis (ATN), no evidence of rejection.

Diagnosis

- Renal thrombotic microangiopathy (TMA). Mesangiolysis is one of the histologic feature of TMA seen in Fig. 9.1, intracapillary fragmented RBCs and fibrin tactoids in Fig. 9.3.
- Severe acute tubular necrosis (ATN).
- No microscopic or molecular evidence of rejection or alloimmune reaction (Figs. 9.2 and 9.3).

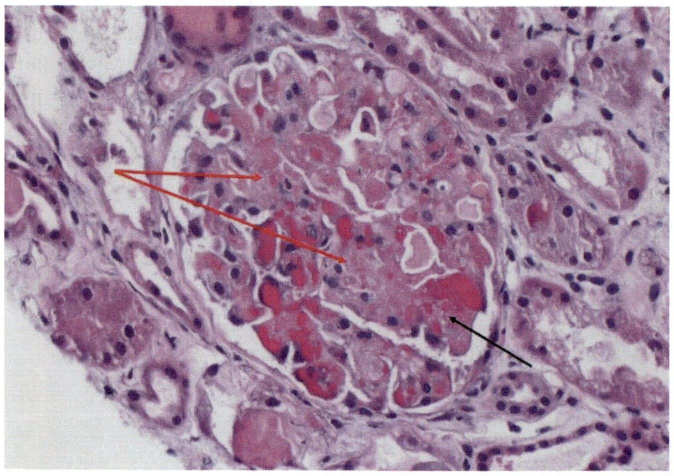

Fig. 9.1 Mesangiolysis as a histologic feature of TMA, (red arrows) and fragmented RBCs (black arrow). H&E 40×

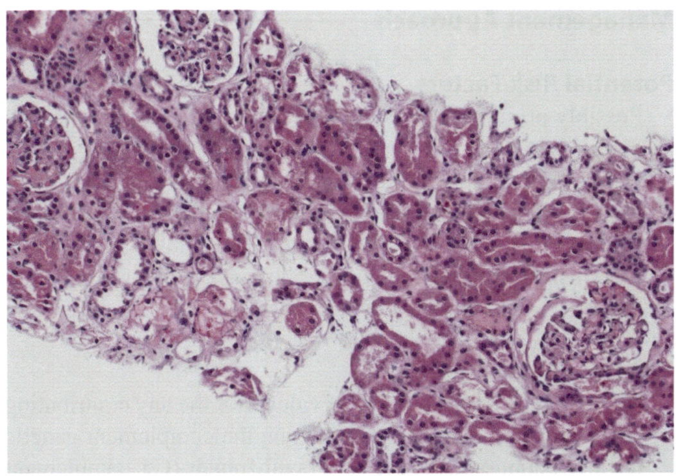

Fig. 9.2 No clear evidence of interstitial inflammation H&E 20×

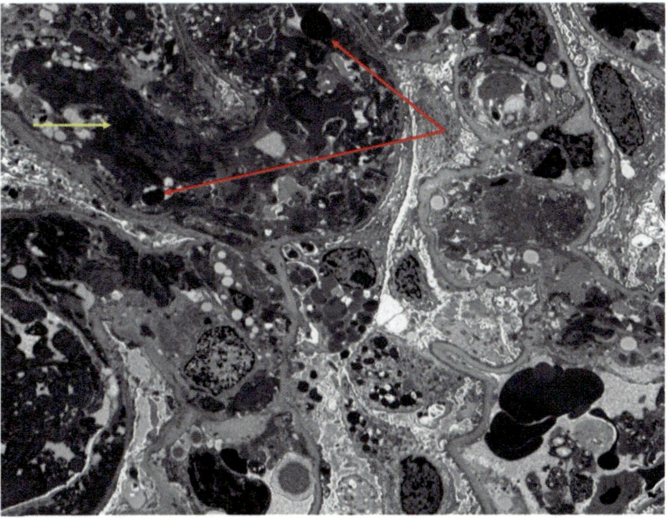

Fig. 9.3 Intracapillary fragmented RBCs (red arrows), and fibrin tactoids (yellow arrow). EM 500×

Management Approach

Potential Risk Factors

- Possibly primary de novo aHUS in the setting of genetic predisposition.
- Potential secondary causes that are not entirely related to this case but require special investigation in other cases including calcineurin inhibitors (CNIs) or mTOR inhibitors, ischemia-reperfusion injury, infection, antibody-mediated rejection (ABMR), and malignant hypertension [1].

Treatment

- Due to the inconclusive direct evidence of the any contributing risk factor and equivocal findings on the complement genetic testing, patient was started on ravulizumab (C5 complement inhibitor) administered for total 6 months.
- Due to high immunologic risk profile patient was kept on tacrolimus-based regimen, maximally tolerated MMF and daily prednisone.

Follow-Up

- Ravulizumab was discontinued after 6 months.
- The patient maintains stable graft function with a serum creatinine of 1.8 mg/dL and no urinary abnormalities for years following his presumptive diagnosis of de novo TMA and complement abnormality.

Educational Insights

- TMA following kidney transplantation is a rare and recognized complication that may become a devastating complication of kidney transplantation.
- In patients with de novo diagnosis of TMA, a systemic workup is critical to exclude other causes (e.g., TTP, aHUS, infection, or drug toxicity).

- Studies show that secondary TMA causes account for most of the presentations, including pregnancy, malignancy, infections, medications, autoimmune diseases, and transplantation process itself [2].
- According to one study a cause was identified in 500 out of 564 patients with TMA diagnosis in all kidney cases (a non transplant cohort): pregnancy (35%), malignancies (19%), infections (33%), drugs (26%), transplantations (17%), autoimmune diseases (9%), shiga toxin due to *Escherichia coli* (6%), and malignant hypertension (4%). While 6% were identified to have a primary cause TTP, and a HUS.
- Identification of genetic variants may support a primary TMA diagnosis, though variants of uncertain significance (VUS) should be interpreted cautiously.
- Complement blockade (e.g., ravulizumab or eculizumab) may be effective in selected cases with suspected complement-mediated TMA.

Pearl 9.1

Thrombotic microangiopathy (TMA) after kidney transplant is rare, and most of the cases following solid organ transplant is secondary or of multifaceted etiologies. A thorough workup is essential to differentiate between primary complement-mediated TMA and secondary causes and complement inhibition can be effective in select cases of both conditions.

Case 9.2

Case Study Summary

Patient: A 42-year-old male with ESRD of unknown etiology who previously lost his first kidney transplant due to rejection.

Transplant course: He underwent a second deceased donor kidney transplant. The patient was sensitized, placing him at higher immunologic risk. He received ATG at 6 mg/kg and steroids for induction and kept on Tac-MMF combination treatment in addition to daily prednisone.

Post-transplant course: The early post-transplant period was complicated by delayed graft function (DGF) and clinical features consistent with microangiopathic hemolytic anemia (MAHA), including:

- Persistent elevated lactate dehydrogenase (LDH), positive schistocytes on peripheral smear.
- ADAMTS13 activity at 56% (non-diagnostic for TTP).
- Normal coagulation parameters (PT/PTT).
- Complement studies including factors H, I, B, and factor H autoantibodies were within normal ranges. A genetic panel for atypical HUS (aHUS) returned equivocal. Serum C5b-9 level was low.
- Negative donor-specific antibodies (DSA).
- Kidney biopsy confirmed pathological thrombotic microangiopathy (TMA) and acute tubular necrosis (ATN).

Diagnosis

- Renal-limited thrombotic microangiopathy (TMA) as seen in (Figs. 9.4 and 9.5).
- Acute tubular necrosis (ATN).

Management Approach

Potential Risk Factors

- Extensive evaluation ruled out TTP, infection, antiphospholipid syndrome (APLS) and other autoimmune disorders, rejection, and primary complement disorder.
- TMA was likely secondary to transplant-related stressors (e.g., ischemia-reperfusion injury, immunologic burden), though a definitive trigger was not identified.

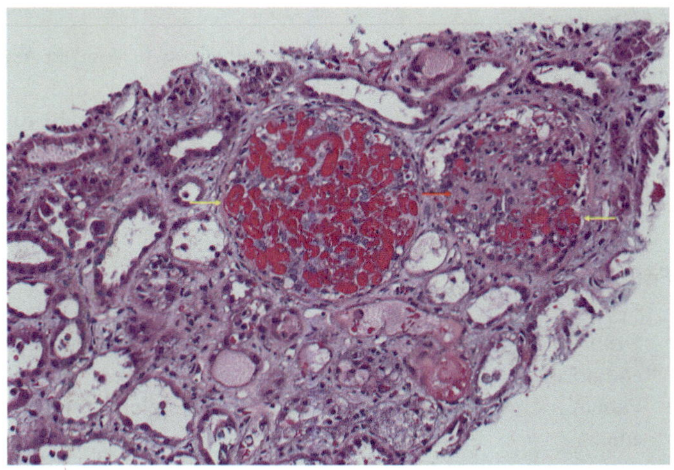

Fig. 9.4 Glomerular capillary stasis, glomerular paralysis (yellow arrows), and mesangiolysis (red arrow) H&E, 20×

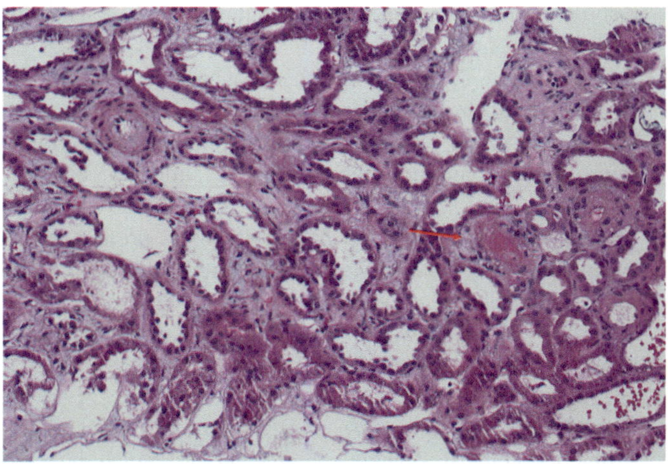

Fig. 9.5 Fibrinoid necrosis and myxoid endothelial hyperplasia of the intralobular arteries (red arrow) H&E, 20×

Treatment

- Initial plasmapheresis (PLEX) × 2 with fresh frozen plasma (FFP) while the diagnostic work up was underway.
- Initiated C5 complement inhibitor therapy (ravulizumab) for 6 months (based on possible VUS of genetic work up and excluding other secondary causes).

Follow-Up

- Graft function remains stable, with inactive urinary sediment and no signs of recurrent TMA.
- Patient responded clinically to PLEX and complement blockade.

Educational Insights

- Thrombotic microangiopathies (TMAs) are a diverse group of disorders that are characterized by common clinical and laboratory features.
- Post-transplant TMA can be either recurrent primary disease (e.g., complement-mediated aHUS, TTP) or de novo, triggered by surgical stress, ischemia-reperfusion injury after kidney transplantation, immunosuppressive drugs, infection, or rejection.
- In patients with atypical or incomplete TMA profiles, a full complement and genetic workup is essential, although results may be inconclusive and need to be interpreted carefully.
- Deferring PLEX may be appropriate in clinically stable patients when alternative diagnoses are more likely than TTP or primary TMA [3].
- Complement inhibition (e.g., ravulizumab) is a rational therapeutic option in cases where complement dysregulation is suspected, even in the absence of a definitive genetic diagnosis [4, 5].

 **Pearl 9.2**

Post-transplant thrombotic microangiopathy (TMA) can occur in the absence of a clear trigger or definitive diagnosis; when primary TMA is suspected but unconfirmed, complement blockade may still be beneficial, particularly in high-risk patients with biopsy-proven TMA and incomplete systemic features.

Case 9.3

Case Study Summary

Patient: A 24-year-old female with end-stage renal disease (ESRD) of unknown etiology.

Transplant: She received a deceased donor kidney transplant (DDKT) from a donor after cardiac death (DCD). She was sensitized (cPRA 37%). She received ATG and steroids for induction, followed by traditional triple immunosuppression treatment of daily prednisone and combination of Tac-MMF.

Post-transplant course: soon after discharge, the patient presented with fever, vomiting, leukocytosis, and worsening hypertension. Doppler ultrasound demonstrated absent flow in the main renal artery and vein renal scintigraphy showed total photopenia, indicating no perfusion or function. These findings prompted an urgent transplant nephrectomy.

Diagnosis

- Infarcted renal allograft with extensive coagulative and hemorrhagic necrosis (Figs. 9.6 and 9.7).
- Complete thrombotic occlusion of both renal artery and vein.

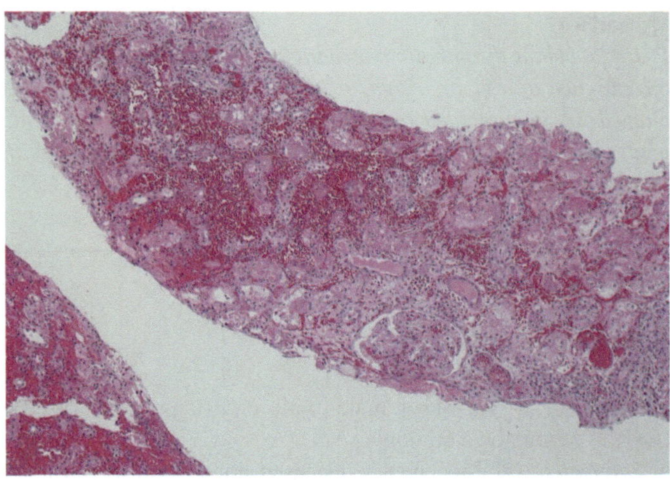

Fig. 9.6 Parenchymal infarction with coagulative and hemorrhagic necrosis on core needle bx specimen, H&E, 10×

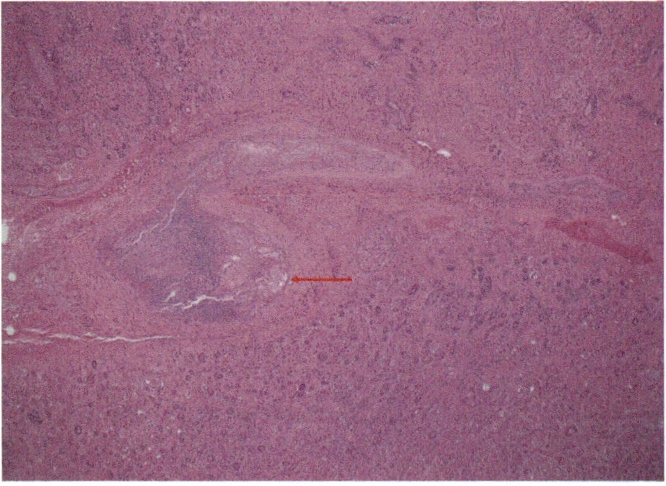

Fig. 9.7 Parenchymal infarction with coagulative necrosis and arterial recent thrombus (red arrow) in the allograft nephrectomy specimen, H&E, 40×

Management Approach

Triggering risk factors: No known historical or current hypercoagulable disorder, no known clinical or molecular evidence of alloimmune activity, no known serological evidence of autoimmune disorders.

Treatment: Transplant nephrectomy.

Follow-Up

The patient returned to dialysis, marked as graft failure.

Educational Insights

- Primary nonfunction (PNF) in renal allograft is a recognized but relatively rare and an uncommon cause of early graft loss, typically occurring within the first 10 days post-transplant.
- Etiologies are often unidentified but may include [6]:
  - Thromboembolism from cardiac or vascular sources.
  - In situ thrombosis due to surgical trauma or anatomic anomalies.
  - Hypercoagulable states (inherited or acquired).
- The pathogenesis is multifactorial, often involving a combination of vascular injury and a prothrombotic environment.
- There is no effective treatment for primary nonfunction (PNF) due to infarction; prevention is key:
  - Careful donor-recipient matching.
  - Thorough hypercoagulable and immunologic workup.
  - Judicious perioperative anticoagulation.

Pearl 9.3

Renal allograft infarction is a rare but devastating cause of early graft loss; it often presents abruptly within days after transplant, and prevention through careful surgical technique, vascular assessment, and hypercoagulability screening is critical, as there is no effective treatment once infarction occurs.

References

1. Imanifard Z. TMA in kidney transplantation. Transplantation. 2023;107(11):2329–40.
2. Bayer G. Etiology and outcomes of thrombotic Microangiopathies. Clin J Am Soc Nephrol. 2019;14(4):557–66. https://doi.org/10.2215/CJN.11470918.
3. Winters JL. Plasma exchange in thrombotic microangiopathies (TMAs) other than thrombotic thrombocytopenic purpura (TTP). Am Soc Hematol. 2017;2017(1):632–8. https://doi.org/10.1182/asheducation-2017.1.632.
4. Golshayan D. Targeting the complement Pathway in Kidney transplantation. J Am Soc Nephrol. 2023;34(11):1776–92. https://doi.org/10.1681/ASN.0000000000000192.
5. Tatapudi VS. Therapeutic modulation of the complement system in kidney transplantation: clinical indications and emerging drug leads. Front Immunol. 2019;10:2306. https://doi.org/10.3389/fimmu.2019.02306.
6. Bakir N. Primary renal graft thrombosis. Nephrol Dial Transplant. 1996;11(1):140–7.

Post-transplant Monoclonal Gammopathy-Related Kidney Injury

10

Hasan Fattah

Case 10.1

Case Study Summary

Patient: A 57-year-old female with end-stage renal disease (ESRD) due to autosomal dominant polycystic kidney disease (ADPKD).

Transplant course: She received a deceased donor kidney transplant (DDKT) and induction treatment with ATG and steroids. Post-transplant course was initially unremarkable with stable graft function.

Clinical course: Five years post-transplant, the patient developed new-onset nephrotic-range proteinuria repeated random UPCR 5–6 g/g with stable serum creatinine at 0.9 mg/dL.

Other Workup

- Donor-specific antibodies (DSA) and donor-derived cell-free DNA (dd-cfDNA): undatable.
- Serum immunofixation (SIF): Faint monoclonal kappa band.

H. Fattah (✉)
Jacob School of Medicine and Biomedical Science,
University at Buffalo, Buffalo, NY, USA

- Urine immunofixation (UIF): negative.
- Kappa/lambda ratio: Elevated at 280 (kappa 1400 mg/L, lambda 5 mg/L).
- Bone marrow biopsy: 18% monoclonal plasma cells, positive for CD38, CD56, CD117, and kappa light chain restriction.
- Kidney biopsy: Confirmed kappa light chain deposition disease (LCDD) with nodular glomerulosclerosis pattern.

Diagnosis

De novo monoclonal immunoglobulin deposition disease (MIDD); kappa light chain type, as seen by increased mesangial matrix with nodular formation under H&E (Fig. 10.1); and positive kappa light chain in (Figs. 10.2 and 10.3a).

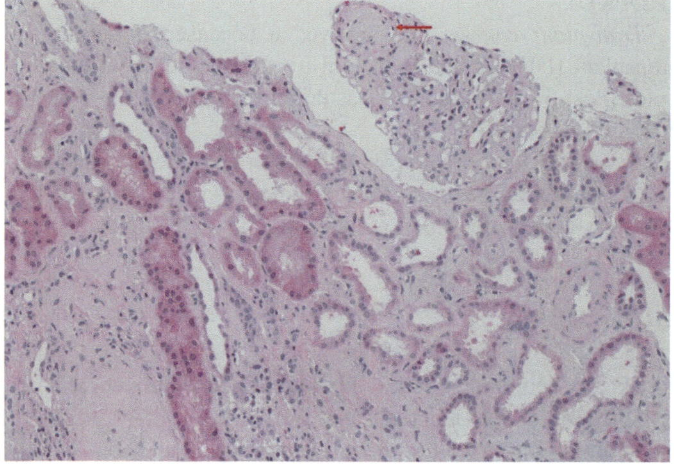

Fig. 10.1 Increased mesangial matrix with nodular formation (red arrow) H&E, 20×

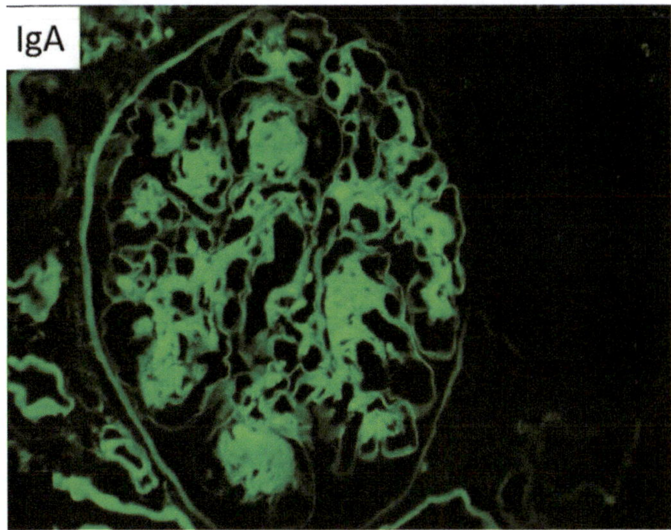

Fig. 10.2 IgA positive staining in the GBM, mesangial areas, Bowman's capsule, and tubular basement membrane. IF for IgA, 20×

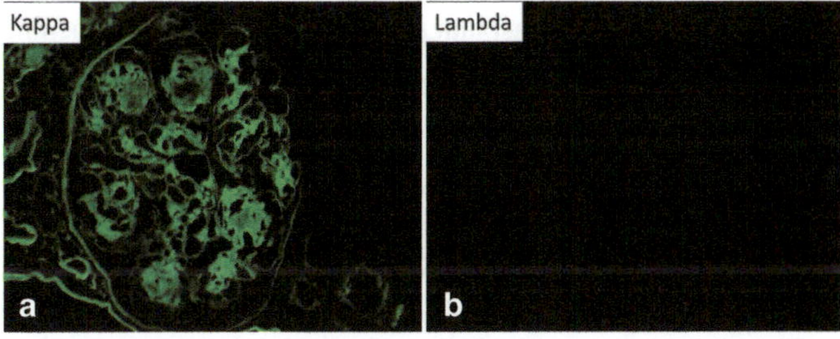

Fig. 10.3 Positive kappa light chain in picture **a**, and negative staining for lambda light chain in picture **b**, IF, 20×

Management Approach

Transplant risk factors: Unrelated to transplantation; considered a de novo plasma cell dyscrasia.

Treatment: Initiated bortezomib and lenalidomide.

Follow-Up

- Proteinuria resolved and serum kappa light chain levels improved with therapy.
- Unfortunately, the patient later developed high-grade disseminated neuroendocrine tumor (NET), treated with capecitabine and temozolomide, and eventually passed away from disease complications.
- The kidney allograft remained functional until death, 5 years after the MIDD diagnosis.

Educational Insights

- De novo monoclonal immunoglobulin deposition disease can occur after kidney transplant but is rare. Most cases happening after kidney transplant are recurrences of the original disease.
- Unlike recurrent disease, de novo cases may occur without detectable serum or urine paraprotein and without evidence of a systemic plasma cell or B-cell clone [1, 2].
- Usually characterized by IgG3 with κ or λ light chain deposition in glomeruli with a membranoproliferative or mesangioproliferative pattern on histology.
- The clinical course is variable, but graft outcomes are generally poor if not promptly recognized and treated [3].

Pearl 10.1

De novo *MIDD should be considered in the differential diagnosis of new-onset glomerular disease in the allograft, even in the absence of a detectable monoclonal gammopathy, high index of suspicion is required for diagnosis.*

Case 10.2

Case Study Summary

Patient: A 62-year-old male with end-stage renal disease (ESRD) secondary to hypertension.

Transplant: He received a living kidney transplant (LKT), thymoglobulin, and steroid induction and maintained on traditional triple immunosuppression composed of daily prednisone and CNI-MMF combination.

Clinical course: Two years post-transplant, the patient developed new-onset nephrotic syndrome, random repeated UPCR 10 g/g; serum albumin, decreased to 2 g/dl; serum creatinine, increased from baseline 1.5 to 2.0 mg/dL, DSA and dd-cfDNA were undetectable; serologic workup, normal except for monoclonal lambda light chain detected on immunofixation electrophoresis; free light chains: lambda: 7094 mg/L; kappa, 13 mg/L; and kappa/lambda ratio, close to 0. Bone marrow biopsy: revealed >60% monoclonal plasma cells, consistent with multiple myeloma (MM).

Kidney involvement: Confirmed monoclonal lambda light chain deposition disease.

Diagnosis

De novo multiple myeloma with monoclonal lambda light chain-mediated; light chain proximal tubulopathy (LCPT), seen as ATN (Fig. 10.4) and positive intracytoplasmic lambda light chain of the cortical tubular epithelial cells (Fig. 10.5).

Management Approach

Transplant risk factors: the Disease is considered unrelated to transplantation, reflecting a de novo plasma cell dyscrasia.

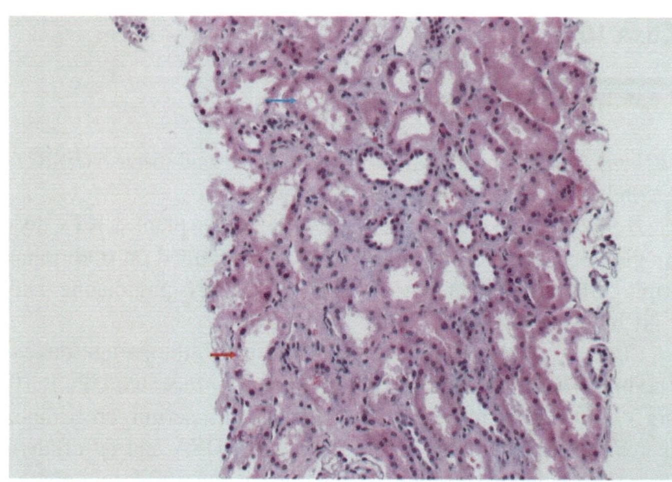

Fig. 10.4 ATN most consistent with light chain proximal tubulopathy (LCPT); epithelial simplification (red arrow) and sloughing off the apical borders of the epithelial cells consistent (blue arrow) with ATN. H&E 20×

Fig. 10.5 Lambda light chain intracytoplasmic staining of the cortical tubular epithelial cells. Immunofluorescence, 20×

Treatment:

- Initiated induction chemotherapy.
- MMF was discontinued; to avoid excessive bone marrow suppression effect, patient was continued on tacrolimus and prednisone only.

Follow-Up

- The patient showed excellent hematologic and renal response to therapy, his paraproteinemia improved, creatinine decreased back to normal baseline, and proteinuria has resolved, unfortunately patient passed away due to acute hypoxic respiratory failure from COVID-19 complication.
- Graft function remained stable until death.

Educational Insights

- Monoclonal gammopathy of renal significance (MGRS) may first present as post-transplant nephrotic syndrome, even in previously stable graft recipients.
- De novo plasma cell neoplasia, such as multiple myeloma, can significantly impact both recipient and graft survival [4, 5].
- The severity of renal involvement and long-term outcomes correlate closely with the hematologic response to chemotherapy.
- Response typically defined by a > 90% reduction in involved free light chain or normalization of serum monoclonal protein—has been shown to be the minimum threshold required for preservation of kidney function and reduction in recurrence risk after transplantation [6].
- Post-transplant proteinuria is independently associated with worse graft and patient outcomes, including higher cardiovascular risk, with risk rising in proportion to the degree of proteinuria [7].

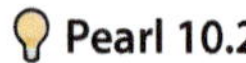

Pearl 10.2

The medical literature consistently demonstrates that de novo *plasma cell disorders after kidney transplantation are associated with high rates of graft loss and patient mortality due to both hematologic progression and infectious complications.*

Case 10.3

Special thanks to Dr. John Tomaszewski for kindly providing case images that helped bring this subject to life.

Case Study Summary

Patient: A 44 year-old male with end-stage renal disease (ESRD) secondary to biopsy-proven membranoproliferative glomerulonephritis MPGN type II per patient past medical history report, associated with C3 nephritic factor (elevated at 0.45 pre-transplant).

Transplant: He received a DDKT, thymoglobulin, and steroid induction and maintained on traditional triple immunosuppression composed of daily prednisone and CNI-MMF combination.

Clinical course: Early course was complicated by delayed graft function, persistent hematuria, and mild proteinuria. This necessitated a kidney biopsy and an extensive serology workup.

- *Pathology*: Confirmed recurrent C3 glomerulonephritis (C3GN), Immunofluorescence was performed on formalin-fixed, paraffin-embedded tissue after pronase digestion to rule out masked monoclonal immunoglobulin deposits.
- *Other Serologies*: Negative DSA, low complements level, elevated kappa/lambda ratio 10.5 by serum free light chain assay, serum protein electrophoresis (SPEP) interpreted as possible monoclonal component seen as an extended band in the beta

region, urine protein electrophoresis (UPEP) revealed monoclonal component in the gamma region, and IFE showed monoclonal IgG kappa migrating in beta region without a corresponding M-spike on SPE; furthermore hematologic evaluation with bone marrow biopsy revealed no evidence of multiple myeloma; thus the diagnosis of monoclonal gammopathy of renal significance (MGRS) was formatted.

- *Genetic evaluation*: Evaluation of 15 genes associated with CM-TMA/a HUS or C3G failed to reveal any pathogenic variants or even variants of uncertain significance (VUS).
- *Clinical conclusion*: Recurrent C3GN likely driven by immune-mediated mechanisms in association with monoclonal gammopathy; other etiologies such as AMR, infectious, and genetic high-risk traits were less likely ones based on negative serology and pathology workup.

Diagnosis

Early recurrent C3 glomerulonephritis (C3GN) associated with monoclonal gammopathy (IgG kappa), no overt diagnosis of plasma cell dyscrasia. Seen as membranoproliferative pattern of glomerular injury in (Fig. 10.6). Immunofluorescence showed exclusive glomerular granular C3 deposition (3–4+) with no labeling for IgG, IgA, or IgM in Fig. 10.7 and subendothelial electron dense deposits under EM in Fig. 10.8.

Management Approach

Transplant risk factors: History of MPGN type II, hypocomplementemia and known history of pre-transplant positive C3 nephritic factor which is a known autoantibody that stabilizes and increase activity of C3 convertase and eventually sustained activation of the alternative complement pathway.

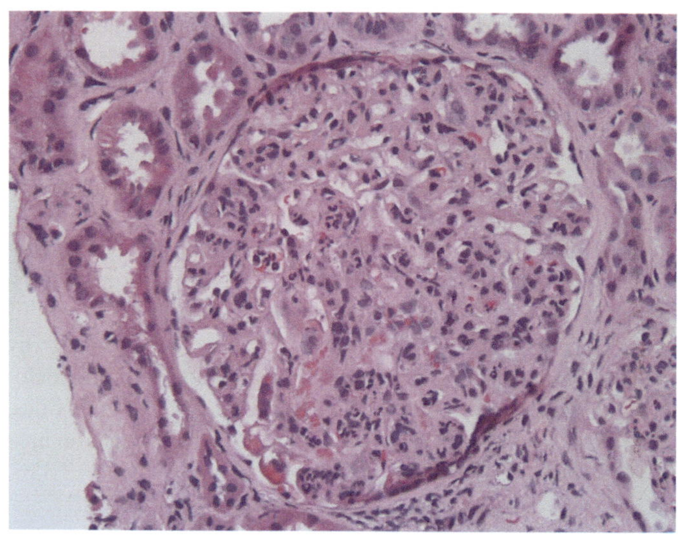

Fig. 10.6 Membranoproliferative pattern of glomerular injury secondary to C3GN, a diffuse mesangial hypercellularity and increased matrix expansion H&E, 40×

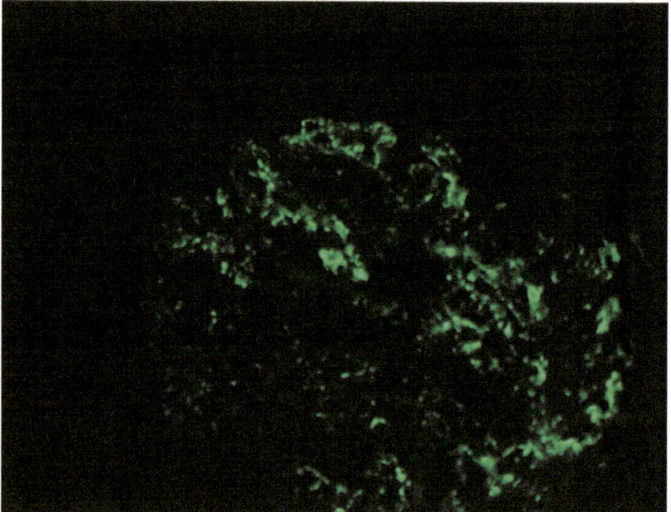

Fig. 10.7 Immunofluorescence shows exclusive glomerular granular C3 deposition (3–4+) with negative staining for IgG, IgA, or IgM. The C3 labeling appears to include both capillary loop and mesangial compartments

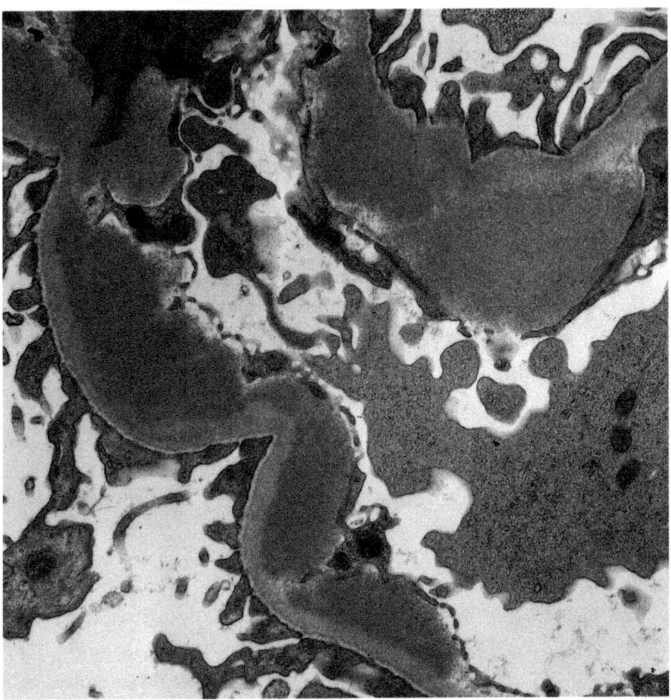

Fig. 10.8 EM with sub-endothelial electron dense deposits 12,000×

Treatment

- Patient received PLEX and steroids and was kept on higher doses of CNI-MMF combination to abate the ongoing autoimmune activity.
- He eventually started on chemotherapy which he received for 6 months consisted of daratumumab *(discontinued later due to intolerance)*, dexamethasone, bortezomib, and cyclophosphamide.

Follow-Up

- The patient showed slow hematologic and renal improvement, both of his proteinuria and hematuria resolved; his renal graft function was stable with new CKD 3b.

Educational Insights

- MPGN is a pattern of glomerular injury, and not a specific disease.
- Classification has changed over time and is best described based on the pathogenetic process, whether it is mediated by immune complexes, monoclonal immunoglobulins, or complement dysregulation.
- According to (KDIGO) guideline, the recurrence risk of C3G is high: about 70% in C3GN and 50–100% in DDD [8].
- Adult series report recurrence in 67% of C3GN with median 14–28 months to recurrence and substantial graft loss attributable to recurrence [9]. More recent protocol-biopsy studies show even higher early subclinical recurrence, with 89% detected within weeks to months, though short-term graft function may be preserved [10].

Pearl 10.3

C3GN is a rare form of glomerulonephritis; it is associated with high risk of recurrence after kidney transplant and sometimes with monoclonal gammopathy; in such cases further hematology evaluation is required to rule out plasma cell dyscrasia and other end-organ involvement.

References

1. Albawardi A. Proliferative glomerulonephritis with monoclonal IgG deposits recurs or may develop De Novo in kidney allografts. Am J Kidney Dis. 2011;58(2):276–81. https://doi.org/10.1053/j.ajkd.2011.05.003.
2. Bridoux F. Proliferative glomerulonephritis with monoclonal immunoglobulin deposits: a nephrologist perspective. Nephrol Dial Transplant. 2021;36(2):208–15. https://doi.org/10.1093/ndt/gfz176.
3. Kamal J. Clinicopathologic assessment of monoclonal immunoglobulin-associated renal disease in the kidney allograft: a retrospective study and review of the literature. Transplantation. 2020;104(7):1341–9. https://doi.org/10.1097/TP.0000000000003010.

4. Kormann R. Plasma cell neoplasia after kidney transplantation: french cohort series and review of the literature. PLoS One. 2017;12(6):e0179406. https://doi.org/10.1371/journal.pone.0179406.
5. Ng JH. Outcomes of kidney transplantation in patients with myeloma and amyloidosis in the USA. Nephrol Dial Transplant. 2022;37(12):2569–80. https://doi.org/10.1093/ndt/gfac196.
6. Leung N. Monoclonal Gammopathy of renal significance. N Engl J Med. 2021;384(20):1931–41. https://doi.org/10.1056/NEJMra1810907.
7. Tsampalieros A. Evaluation and management of proteinuria after kidney transplantation. Transplantation. 2015;99(10):2049–60. https://doi.org/10.1097/TP.0000000000000894.
8. Chadban SJ, et al. KDIGO clinical practice guideline on the evaluation and management of candidates for kidney transplantation. Transplantation. 2020;104(4S1):S11–S103.
9. Zand L. Clinical findings, pathology, and outcomes of C3GN after kidney transplantation. JASN. 2014;25(5):1110–7. https://doi.org/10.1681/ASN.2013070715.
10. Tarragón B. C3 glomerulopathy recurs early after kidney transplantation in serial biopsies performed within the first 2 years after transplantation. Clin J Am Soc Nephrol. 2024;19(8):1005–15. https://doi.org/10.2215/CJN.0000000000000474.

Index

H. Fattah, V. Cornea (eds.), *Transplantation in Practice*,
https://doi.org/10.1007/978-3-032-15908-3

GPSR Compliance

The European Union's (EU) General Product Safety Regulation (GPSR) is a set of rules that requires consumer products to be safe and our obligations to ensure this.

If you have any concerns about our products, you can contact us on ProductSafety@springernature.com

In case Publisher is established outside the EU, the EU authorized representative is:

Springer Nature Customer Service Center GmbH
Europaplatz 3
69115 Heidelberg, Germany

Batch number: 10370710

Printed by Printforce, the Netherlands